MIMESIS
INTERNATIONAL

PHILOSOPHY
n. 48

DISRUPTION OF HABITS DURING THE PANDEMIC

Edited by
Corinna Guerra and Marco Piazza

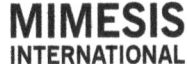
MIMESIS
INTERNATIONAL

This volume is published with the support of the Department of Philosophy, Communication and Performing Arts of the Roma Tre University, in the frame of "The Public Dynamics of Fear and Inclusive Citizenship" Project, funded by the Roma Tre University, under Action 4: "Experimental action to finance innovative and interdisciplinary research projects".

CONTENTS

CORINNA GUERRA, MARCO PIAZZA

INTRODUCTION

1. *February 2020: the global disruption*

A leading characteristic of any pandemic is that its history is expressed in numbers.[1] The purpose of this book is precisely to analyse the 2019 Coronavirus (COVID-19) pandemic beyond its numbers.

Rather, the authors focus on the impact of the pandemic on people's habits, ranging from the individual to the social. That our ways of navigating daily life and surviving in this world were so profoundly disrupted by the pandemic has proved to be a truly stimulating research topic for philosophers and historians.

The chronicle of past pandemics is rich in testimonies on the drama of the abandonment of habits and rituals that mark the daily life of individuals and their communities. For example, one of the rituals that in normal times, in every age, is part of the social customs is that connected to the death of a relative or a family member. Throughout the plague epidemics that devastated Europe between 1348 and 1720, one of the most destabilizing circumstances was the impossibility of burying the dead according to religious rites. Death became so indecent, so desacralized, so anonymous and repulsive, that it plunged entire populations into despair until they risked madness; suddenly they had been deprived of the spiritual practices that in grief provide dignity, security and identity to individuals. In the chronicles one finds evidence of the joy of the inhabitants of Marseilles, when, at the end of the epidemic of 1720, they saw the funeral carriages reappear in the streets, a sign that the dead were again being buried according to common rites.[2]

---

1   See the chapter by David Vincent in this book. This paragraph is a joint work of Corinna Guerra and Marco Piazza. Paragraph 2 is attributed to Marco Piazza and paragraph 3 to Corinna Guerra.

2   Charles Carrière, Marcel Courdurie, and Ferréol Rebuffat, *Marseille, ville morte: la peste de 1720* (Marseille: M. Garçon, 1968), p. 124.

Italians will recall watching the events of Bergamo from their televisions: the horrific parade of military trucks carrying the coffins of the dead far outside the city because there was no more space in its mortuaries or cemeteries, preventing family members from any form of recollection on the coffins of their dead relatives and from celebrating funerals. As with the current pandemic, the overturning of habits was total: productive activities stopped, the cities fell in silence, the sick were isolated and came to find themselves in complete solitude, death was shrouded in anonymity, and collective rites were abolished, both those of joy and amusement and those of prayer and pain.

This abrupt and brutal suspension of habits, both then and now, was accompanied by an almost total impossibility to formulate plans for the future. In times of crisis, therefore, there is a crisis in the perception of time: the epidemic obliges us to consider every minute as a simple delay and to have no other perspective in front of us than that of probable, imminent death. As Jean Delumeau, author of a masterly history of fear in the West, stresses, "by disrupting common structures and preventing any project for the future", the pandemic "in this way disrupted doubly the psychic foundations both individual and collective".[3]

Since World War II, much of the world has entered in *the age of anxiety*[4], a recurring element in public discourse and private life spread by processes of globalization. Many writers and historians have focused this prevalent approach to life since at least the twentieth century, but a debate has been rekindled following the terrorist attacks of the 2000s.

In France in particular, after the Bataclan massacre of November 13th, 2015, scholars began to consider whether, to quote a verse from the immortal poet Wystan H. Auden, "Then back they come, the fears we fear".[5] No epoch is without fear, but such global events unleash a sort of collective fear linked with incertitude, or anxiety. In many ways, terrorist attacks and the COVID-19 pandemic feed the same kind of anxiety: one

---

3   Jean Delumeau, *La peur en Occident (XIVe-XVIIIe siècles). Une cité assiégée* (Paris: Fayard, 1978), p. 130.

4   Wystan H. Auden, *The Age of Anxiety* (London: Faber & Faber, 1948).

5   Guerra is very grateful to Jean-Jacques Courtine for letting her read the unpublished text of his conference *La peur à l'age de l'anxiété, histoire d'une émotion contemporaine* given in Lausanne, October 20th, 2017, at the Dorigny University Campus, to which many of the following considerations belong to. Jean-Jacques Courtine, Alain Corbin, Georges Vigarello, *Histoire des émotions. De la fin du XIXe siècle à nos jours* (Paris: Seuil, 2017), vol. 3, ch. on Anxiety. Auden, p. 24. William G. Naghy and Penny Roberts, *Fear in Early Modern Society* (Manchester: Manchester University Press, 1997).

linked with social life, with activities that we share with other human beings. More importantly, these events disrupt our habits as individuals and as groups. This is not to say that in the past people did not have anxiety; indeed, they feared famines and epidemics, but such events were limited within a perimeter or territory. Instead, anxiety is now linked to a globalized world: global fear, individual anxiety. Anyone could testify that anxiety grew over SARS-CoV-2 due to the highly interconnected world we live in. We now face a future of pandemic, just as 20 years ago we learned to face a future of terrorist attacks. In this context, fear itself seems to be a habit.

However, putting aside similarities, one major difference remains, and it is connected with the limitations of our individual freedom, but all of these points will be discussed in the following book chapters.

These are only some of the issues that we kept in mind when looking for scholars to involve in the webinar *Fear and Disruption of habits during the global pandemic*, which is at the origin of this volume, and we wish that the contributions and resulting discussions will produce an historical and philosophical gaze on what we are experiencing, and a better grasp on our future.

2. *Disruption of habits*

Western philosophy has involved itself since Aristotle in the explanation of the formation of habits and customs, and over the centuries has proposed a series of models to explain them by first dialoguing with medical knowledge and more recently with anthropology, psychology and sociology.[6] Around the mid-nineteenth century, one of the greatest scholars of habit, Félix Ravaisson, in describing the un-reflexive spontaneity that marks habits in the sphere of sensations and emotions, wrote of a need and a desire that settles within us without our realizing it.[7] Other philosophers, like Maine de Biran and the novelist Marcel Proust, also dwelled on this

---

6   Tom Sparrow and Adam Hutchinson (eds.), *A History of Habit. From Aristotle to Bourdieu* (Lanham: Lexington Books, 2013); Clare Carlisle, *On Habit* (London: Routledge, 2014); Marco Piazza, *Creature dell'abitudine. Abito, costume, seconda natura da Aristotele alle scienze cognitive* (Bologna: Il Mulino, 2018).

7   Félix Ravaisson, *De l'habitude* (Paris: Fournier, 1838), transl. by Clare Carlisle and Mark Sinclair, *Of Habit* (London: Continuum, 2008).

sense of addiction generated by habit.[8] They show that the feeling reveals itself when a habit is interrupted in a sudden and traumatic way; a kind of interruption that causes pain and anguish. It is at this point that we realize, Proust says, how the habit is a "divinité redoutable" (*dread deity*), and not just a "aménageuse habile" (*skilful arranger*) that helps us adjust to a new environment.[9] An example produced by Proust is that of the trauma that occurs when a loved one abandons us without notice, whether because he flees or because he dies; despite the passion we felt, it had been blunted by habituation, and the abrupt interruption of the ménage produces a very strong pain and a feeling of total disorientation.[10]

In the preparatory work for the Webinar at the origin of this book, we wondered if Western philosophy had tried to reflect on this device of the interruption of habit not only from the point of view of the individual and his passions, but also on a social scale and in relation to collective events. We know that since Plato there has been a conservative line of thought that warns us against the subversion of customs, traditions, and laws.[11] Along this same line, but many centuries later, we see Montaigne, Charron, and Pascal, and we can still find traces of this thought in the work of William James.[12] However, any deep reflection on the traumatic effects caused by the sudden interruption of our social habits is difficult to find before the development of social psychology and sociology at the turn of the twentieth century. There are traces in the work of French philosopher Léon Dumont (often ignored but much appreciated by the already mentioned William James).[13]

---

8   Maine de Biran, *Mémoires sur l'influence de l'habitude*, ed. by Gilbert Romeyer-Dherbey, in *Oeuvres, II*, ed. by François Azouvi (Paris: Vrin, 1987); Marcel Proust, *À la recherche du temps perdu*, ed. by Jean-Yves Tadié, 4 vols (Paris: Gallimard, 1987-1989), vol. I, p. 17, trans. by Charles K. Scott Moncrieff and Terence Kilmartin, revised by Dennis J. Enright, *In Search of Lost Time*, 6 vols (New York: The Modern Library, 1992-1993), I, p. 15.

9   Erika Fülop, 'Habit in "À la recherche du temps perdu"', *French Studies*, 68(3) (2014), 344-58; Marco Piazza, 'Proust, philosophe de l'habitude', *Revue d'études proustiennes*, 5 (2017), 361-76.

10   Marcel Proust, *À la recherche du temps perdu*, vol. III, pp. 772-73, engl. trans., V, pp. 477-78.

11   Plato, *Leg.* 798d.

12   On Montaigne, Charron, and Pascal see: Marco Piazza, *L'antagonista necessario. La filosofia francese dell'abitudine da Montaigne a Deleuze* (Milan: Mimesis, 2015). On James see directly: William James, 'The Laws of Habit', *Popular Science Momthly*, 30 (1887), 433–51, repr. with modifications in: *Principles of Psychology*, 2 vols (New York: Holt, 1890, vol. I, pp. 104–27).

13   On Dumont's life and works see: Alexander Büchner, *Un philosophe amateur. Essai biographique sur Léon Dumont (1837-1877), avec extraits de sa*

Dumont, who in 1876 provided a materialistic interpretation of habit, interprets the history of societies in an evolutionary framework, showing how a traumatic social event tends to be followed by a restoration of past collective habits because old habits retain power for a long time after they are abruptly interrupted.[14] This is demonstrated in history by the restoration of previous political orders following revolutions, and obviously Dumont has here in mind the Restoration that followed the French Revolution of 1789.[15] Another trace can be found in a January 1914 lecture given by one of the fathers of modern sociology, Émile Durkheim. Reflecting on Dewey's pragmatism, Durkheim notes that in the interruption of mechanical habit, reflection takes control again of our acting in a condition of "uncertainty, tension, anxiety".[16] Our efforts in such a situation are all focused on "re-establish[ing] the lost equilibrium", showing how our reflexive activity is therefore not merely 'speculative' but 'primarily practical'.[17]

But what happens when we can't restore the destroyed balance? Generally, thinkers like Dumont or Durkheim argue that we will try to re-establish equilibrium, and that our neuronal and organic plasticity allows us to adapt to the new environment, so much that those who succeed most effectively in this enterprise have the upper from an evolutionary point of view. In some cases, however, the spectre of an impossible restoration of broken equilibrium appears, with the consequent disintegration of the living organism, and its death.[18]

But no one seems to draw on the long history of pandemics or other natural disasters to try to test his theories. The epidemics, especially those of cholera that mark the nineteenth century, left a trace in social psychology on the question of the contagiousness of fear among the masses. In the case of epidemic diseases, for centuries it was believed that the effects of fear

---

correspondence (Paris: Alcan, 1884). On Dumont's theory of habit see: Catherine Dromelet, 'Léon Dumont, Sensibilité, plaisir et habitude', *Revue philosophique*, 4, t. 143 (2018), 479-94; Catherine Dromelet, 'Une science de la sensibilité. Dumont, l'habitude et le plaisir', in L. Dumont, *De l'habitude et du plaisir*, ed. by Catherine Dromelet (Paris: Garnier, 2019), pp. 7–24.

14   Léon Dumont, 'L'Habitude', *Revue philosophique de la France et de l'Étranger*, 1 (1876), 321-66.

15   *Ibid.*, p. 363.

16   Émile Durkheim, *Pragmatisme et sociologie. Cours inédit prononcé à la Sorbonne en 1913-14 et restitué par A. Cavillier d'après les notes d'édtudiants* (Paris: Vrin, 1955), p. 45, transl. by John C. Whitehouse, *Pragmatism and Sociology* (Cambridge: Cambridge University Press, 1983), p. 38.

17   *Ibid.*

18   Dumont, 'L'Habitude', p. 355.

contributed to an increase in the number of patients and deaths.[19] In other words, the viral contagion is associated with an emotional contagion that claims further victims.[20] The roots of this theory go down in the history of medicine, since the time of Paracelsus, who believed that the infected air could not cause the plague alone, but could provoke the disease by combining with the leaven of fear.[21] After all, fear can become a habit itself![22]

In the long history of the study of pandemics, there is no trace, however, of a link between the two terms of the question, that of fear and that of the interruption of habits. We should thus ask ourselves today what knowledge we need to avoid a situation like that generated by the virus SARS-CoV-2, where fear paralyzes us and prevents us from finding a new equilibrium with our habits. And while we are looking for that knowledge, why not also find a new equilibrium that is even better than the one before it?

3. *A way out from disruption*

As already stated, the chapters that follow are the result of the papers and debate that took place in December 2020, still under the pressure to reflect on what was happening to us, to our lives, to our way of being in the world. All the scholars involved in the international webinar and in the writing of this book were asked to give their contribution to this subject of research *in fieri*, on the disruption of habits due to the pandemic that we were still experiencing at the time. It is thus an open book, perhaps one to be continued, but whose contents are nonetheless profoundly rich and human, as we forced ourselves to reason on events and feelings that touched us personally as scholars and as human beings.

Perhaps it remains to be discussed who will take care of the psychological effects caused by the COVID-19 pandemic, as academic research generally focused on people affected by the actual disease caused by the presence of the virus in the body, while a great part of the population was deeply

---

19   Frédéric Charbonneau, *Quarantine and Caress*, in Claire L. Carlin (ed. by), *Imagining Contagion in Early Modern Europe* (New York: Palgrave, 2005), 124–38, p. 126.

20   Jean Delumeau, p. 131.

21   Walter Pagel, *Paracelsus: An Introduction to Philosophical Medicine in the Era of the Renaissance*, 2nd rev. ed. (Basel; New York: Karger, 1982), p. 141.

22   Lars Svendsen, *Frykt* (Oslo: Universitetsforlaget, 2007), trans. by John Irons, *A Philosophy of Fear* (London: Raktion Books, 2008), p. 46.

affected on a psychological level without ever developing the disease. Beyond that, many other topics have been illustrated by the authors of this volume that can be read in more than one way, but we outline some peculiar elements that emerged.

As is already known, what we used to think of as our daily routines have been profoundly disrupted since 2020. The responsible factors are the fear of the expanding global pandemic, which became increasingly real and close in a very short amount of time, as well as the measures introduced in attempts to contain it. These measures were imposed without any preliminary debate, leaving us with no margin for negotiation: suddenly we were deprived of our interactions, which were a fundamental part of our habits.

For centuries, philosophers have reflected on the influence of habit on individual human conduct (especially from a moral perspective). Between the eighteenth and nineteenth centuries, they refined and arrived at a theory that we call the "double law of habit".[23] When they addressed the issue of customs, namely collective habits, these philosophers generally emphasized the caution required when it comes to changing them. Indeed, a society is at risk when its longstanding traditions, passed down through generations, are suddenly replaced with new ones; when that happens, the risk is anarchy. And the seeming advantages of such a mutation are almost always surpassed by the drawbacks. In other terms, the social upheaval represented by anarchy can entail political actions of repression or restoration of order of a violence that is equal if not superior to that of any revolutionary transformation.

---

23 The so-called "double law of habit" was developed apparently independently in the Anglo-Saxon area by Butler and Hume around the middle of the eighteenth century and then, at the turn of the century, in France by Bichat and Maine de Biran. It then found a mature formulation in Félix Ravaisson's famous doctoral thesis *Of Habit* (1838) and was taken up by William James at the end of the nineteenth century, who adapted it to the neurophysiology of his time. This is the law according to which habit, through repetition or exercise, weakens our passive sensations, to which we basically become progressively accustomed, while it strengthens our active judgements. At the same time, however, it removes our reactions, whether motor or mental, from the sphere of attention, making them spontaneous or automatic and therefore easier and less tiring, and thus transforming them into inclinations or tendencies that are however endowed with a certain reversibility. See: Marco Piazza, 'Fasci ambulanti di abitudini', in William James, *Le leggi dell'abitudine* (1887), italian trans. by Denise Vincenti (Milan-Udine: Mimesis, 2019), pp. 61–67.

Basically, whether habits are individual or social, they constitute a neatly woven fabric of daily life, and routines keep human beings bound to their roles and social functions. Habits enable society as a whole to function and evolve, inasmuch as each individual operates therein like an oiled gear in a giant engine.

De Matteis opens the discussion stressing the old and new rituals that involve individuals, families, and ordinary citizens during the first lockdown. According to his text, each society must decide how to face the shock of a pandemic and each component of society—adolescents, for instance – must elaborate its own way of reacting. To maintain a certain civil society equilibrium, De Matteis argues, we must take these questions into consideration. This analysis offers us an insight both on the flaws and on the virtuous mechanisms of the Italian social system and of neighbourly relations, for example, which still exist at a private level in certain Italian towns.

Are we sure that all the routines resulting from lifestyles, consumption habits, and ways of thinking directing the development of a given society are actually and necessarily leading us towards something better? And, do they lead any given society in a direction that safeguards its viability?

Podgorny, again referring to society's vital rituals, asks whether fear and uncertainty produce new objects instead of simply paralysing our common rituals. She recounts a strange situation in which eukaryotic organisms are turned into virus survival machines. This virus, which is jumping between the animal species that preceded us and that will outlive us, according to Podgorny, could be an opportunity for innovation.

What happened to habits in past pandemics? Did they ever become opportunities for innovation? To understand the pandemic, we appreciate a sort of dialectic process between history and memory where the point of reference is always the Plague. Guérios investigates the media's habitual recourse to the plague as a reference for every epidemic of the past, as if there had been no other worrying epidemic in between it and COVID-19. Perhaps it depends on the cyclical nature of the plague outbreaks, which would not fade after a few years but would rather run their course periodically in nearly every generation. This recurrent pattern ensured that the plague would not be ignored or forgotten, and it provides us with a coherent and simple narrative, which is a cultural and psychological need during a frightful pandemic. However, reference to the distant past in the occasion of traumatic events appears to be preferred, although it means we must compare habits that were markedly different from ours.

In fact, today, loneliness is very common – so common that it can be widely diagnosed as a modern "epidemic" or "plague", as quoted by Vincent.

If we pause and reflect on the way we live our days, considering them in minute detail, we are forced to admit, as already highlighted, that our collective habits represent primary points of reference in our lives. In this framework, loneliness is one important characteristic of our society, and it was supposedly becoming more severe throughout the various lockdowns. We obeyed the measures that were supposed to contain the virus but that ultimately affected our mental equilibrium as we were deprived of what makes us human.[24]

Vincent, however, argues that we were not as lonely as first expected: we had far fewer routine activities we could do, which, very interestingly, are often solitary activities.

Among the solitary activities that COVID-19 has certainly brought with it are the digital ones. But it should be recognized, in Petrocelli's opinion, that the pandemic accelerated those phenomena and processes that were slow to start: the so-called *digital transformation*. COVID-19 has in fact disrupted and digitally rebuilt all aspects of our daily life, from sociality to learning and from consumption to entertainment, causing us some inconveniences but, also and above all, great opportunities. As technology has revealed itself a way out from the crisis, Petrocelli sees an opportunity to encourage societies to invest more in its development. On the other hand, if we consider the fates of the plant and animal species that have gone extinct before us, we can legitimately ask whether our consumption rhythms and pre-pandemic, globalized lifestyles — together with the hole in the ozone layer and other man-made environmental catastrophes linked with technology— were not leading to our downfall?

Nonetheless, in this chapter we find that habits and the disruption of them are very dependent on the technology of the time.

---

24 A position in this regard, which deserves our attention, was expressed in a TV show by the art historian Tomaso Montanari. Theatres and museums are what makes us human, he argued, so their prolonged closure constituted a renunciation of being human, with all the psychological discomfort this entails. *Montanari cita Churchill: "Quando gli chiesero di chiudere i teatri disse: Ma allora per che cosa stiamo combattendo?"* He stated "Art is not superfluous at times like these, it allows us to move forward." February 16th, 2021 <https://www.la7.it/coffee-break/video/montanari-cita-churchill-quando-gli-chiesero-di-chiudere-i-teatri-disse-ma-allora-per-che-cosa-16-02-2021-365575> (last access: November 15th, 2021).

The mentioned interactions, real or virtual, used to shape the structure of our days, created the comforting form of our existence. The sudden changes brought about by the pandemic not only tore up our road maps, but vehiculated the feeling that it also violated our freedom of choice. This started a process, as Baggio analyzes in his essay, of incorporating the scientific debate into the political debate, fed by philosophers and intellectuals' reflections on the relationship between political power and individual liberty, and on the role played by the state of emergency in the delicate equilibrium between a free society and a tyrannical one. In this case, the catastrophe would be human, not sanitary.

Then, with Dromelet we explore whether the classic sociologists can be called upon to better understand what happened to our habits linked to rituals, social groups, etc., as personality is deeply involved in the identification with social roles.

Reflecting on identification with social groups, Vincenti pays attention to the natural tendency in human beings to conform to certain collective behaviors, in particular when strong feelings like fear hurt us. Human history is constantly marked by psychological contagions – in the words of Sergi, the 'epidemic psychosis' of groups. They are the powerful drivers of history. This led us to a paradox where, in the era of social distancing and lockdowns, the group seemed to have exerted more influence on the individual than ever. This appears to prove that social isolation does not necessarily mean psychological independence from others.

Individuals' self-psychological integrity is at the centre of the study written by Aiello and Marraffa. Considering the relation between unconscious cognitive processes and self-consciousness, they discuss the social and emotive relationship's role in the construction of the mind.

The disruption of habits weakens the domestic relationship with the world, exposes the frailty of the self, and calls upon it to buffer the disruption as best as it can. In normal conditions, on the other hand, the self-memory system is enough to guarantee biographical continuity to find new habits that make the world familiar again. The COVID-19 pandemic has displayed many social and individual practices of re-domesticating the world and of interpersonal space, as De Matteis also shows. What will be the destiny of the most fragile individuals? As individuals belonging to different groups, they would display different attitudes and patterns of reaction facing crisis as well as different degrees of ontological security, in accordance with their different combinations of defensive endowments.

A combination of different practices seems to be the only exit to the *impasse* of disrupted habits, so Piazza considers plasticity and flexibility in our habit-building as the answer to this crisis. Plasticity could be appreciated also at a different level, if we consider that the pandemic could transform individual habit into group habit due to fear.

A future of fear is obviously not an optimistic scenario, but many scholars are seeing the possibility that pandemics may become quite recurrent. While this hypothesis suggests a catastrophe for our system of habits, there are populations that are accustomed to living with natural risks who don't need to change their habits every time the event takes place. Guerra illustrates a tentative parallel between living in a red zone of volcanic risk and living in a society where pandemics could be recurrent. These populations have negotiated a set of habits with the particular environment they live in: living close to an active volcano is therefore not so different from living in an epoch where an epidemic is impossible to contain.

If we agree that a transformation of habits is a less traumatic exit to this crisis, of course, we may then consider that this pandemic (like many other catastrophic events that shattered daily life) can teach us to rectify our bad habits, thus enabling us to find a type of collective well-being that would be more sustainable. We can start by redefining our concepts of local and global, or of emergency, but above all, as Bensaude-Vincent stresses, it is vital that we negotiate new habits to live in a more sustainable time. In fact, time is the central point that was hit by the coronavirus crisis of 2019-2021, in the sense of our chronological framework. Crisis, according to the author, is the result of a conflict of temporalities, and consequently challenges the notion of a single universal timeline. Bensaude-Vincent encourages the use of a notion of "timescapes", which considers multiple regimes of temporalities of things we interact with, due to the interdependencies created by technological choices.

New crisis, new time, new habits?

Acknowledgments

This volume originates from the International Webinar on "Fear and disruption of habits during the global pandemic" that we organised in the Department of Philosophy, Communication and Performing Arts at Roma Tre University on December 16th-17th, 2020. That initiative, as well as this volume, are part of the research activity of The Public Dynamics of Fear and Inclusive Citizenship Project, funded by Roma Tre University under "Action 4: Experimental action to finance innovative and interdisciplinary research projects"coordinated by Mario De Caro (Roma Tre University). We warmly thank Mario De Caro for supporting this initiative.

Finally, the editors are very grateful to the Maison Suger of the Fondation Maison des sciences de l'homme (FMSH) in Paris: a wonderful place to live, study, and meet colleagues with whom to start brand new projects, such as this book.

Venice-Rome, November 16th, 2021

STEFANO DE MATTEIS

LIVING THE PANDEMIC
Fears, Risks, and Rituals

1. *Let's Start with the Facts*

On March 9th, 2020, Italy stops.[1] Not because of a blackout, but as a result of a governmental decision taken to protect the population from an enemy as invisible as it is elusive: a virus. This containment measure was dragged out until June 3rd.

This first lockdown was like a freeze-frame: everything stopped without a collective awareness of what was going on. However, at least for once, Italy banded together with such a sense of responsibility and cooperation that gained international recognition. The entire country grit their teeth, stayed strong, and everyone, in their own rooms, homes or apartments, made up rituals and pastimes, devised different opportunities to socialise, and tried out new modes of relationality with their close ones. At the same time, they experimented with the 'social' affordances of technological infrastructures — such as Facebook or Instagram — that had, until then, been used exclusively for entertainment purposes – to mend the familial, romantic, or friendship bonds that the pandemic had loosened or severed. Everyone, either separately or in small groups, came up with ideas to 'resist' the unexpected circulation of the SARS-CoV-2 virus.[2]

In the months of March, April, and May 2020, a 'suspension' was created.[3] A void, where several threads were becoming intertwined: a new, uncharted, never previously experienced event, and the concurrent tragedy

---

1 The article I am presenting is the revised version of the essay 'An Uncertain World. Lockdown Between Risks and Rituals', originally published in *Dada. Rivista di antropologia post-globale* in June 2021.

2 See also Stefano De Matteis, 'Fermo immagine, rituali e strategie; come far fronte al lockdown nella vita quotidiana', *Psicoterapia psicoanalitica*, XXVII, 2020(2), 175–93.

3 Francesco Remotti, 'Sospensione, accecamento, Antropocene', in Marco Aime, Adriano Favole, and Francesco Remotti, *Il mondo che avrete. Virus, Antropocene, Rivoluzione* (Milan: Utet, 2020), pp. 19 onwards.

of a large number of deaths. A painful calamity, nevertheless, that was only to be understood through recollections of the Spanish flu; perhaps slightly less arduous for those located far away from its epicenter, that is, outside of the 'red zones' or neither infected nor directly struck by the fatalities; yet much more harrowing if experienced from the perspective of the victims in the more affected areas. Still, for many, this was an experience of discovery, which, albeit rooted in forced reclusion, branched out into new ways to communicate (such as through balconies and patios, either real or virtual, turned into squares, cafes, and communal spaces).

But if the first lockdown was a freeze-frame and a suspension, the second, which started at the end of September, was a fatal hiccup. After having suffered for those first three months, beginning in June we lived through a collective delusion thinking that the reassuring and comfortable slogan launched at the outbreak of the pandemic, "everything will be alright", had finally come true: it was possible to roam around on bikes and electric scooters purchased with the help of generously issued state subsidies, and even to book a holiday partially granted by government incentives to jump-start the economy.

Everything gave the impression that, at least in Italy, we were on our way back to 'normal'. Sure, the news was not always uplifting, a set-back, a second wave, was hinted at, but October seemed far away. And so was danger. And this enabled people's *carpe diem* (seize the day) attitude.

In June, July, August, September everyone was striving to invigorate the economy, win their *loisir* (leisure) back, and make up for lost time with recreational and entertainment activities, with friends, in public squares, at the seaside.

At the end of September, things got complicated. Or rather, things had never gotten any easier, but there they were, bouncing back with all their tragic potential: the disease spreading like wildfire, its variants multiplying, the death toll increasing. An unexpected crisis for those who fooled themselves into thinking that everything was over. From that moment, Italy is subject to partial and intermittent lockdowns: Italian people are victims of continuous openings and closings, a relentless stop and go that led to despair.[4] The summer months had not been sufficient to rebuild a dwindling economy, one already put to the test and weakened by the first pandemic-induced 'blackout'. For many, it was like standing on the brink of the abyss.

---

4   On these topics, see also Luca Ricolfi, *La notte delle ninfee. Come si malgoverna un'epidemia* (Milan: La nave di Teseo, 2021).

Let's look at this second lockdown a little closer. And let's walk through it following different leads that will help us structure an overview, however provisional, since we are all still in the midst of the storm.

2. General Characters

In this second phase, two burdensome, closely related, causes of uncertainty have been identified in Europe, and, in particular, in Italy. The first one is 'institutional', and it concerns the way the government has handled the pandemic, often by giving contradictory indications (like holiday bonus, or cashback government incentives, countered by partial lockdowns, announced-yet-not-counteracted risk of infection...). The second one concerns the citizens, who were confused by these conflicting signs, and unable to imagine neither solutions nor alternatives.

The 'public' response has been very diverse, depending on the area and the rules enforced therein. Often, however, the most encountered behaviours, regardless of geographical origin, were attempts at 'normality', which were implemented even in violation of the established rules: breaking curfew, visiting friends and family, flocking the streets, chasing happy hours, going back to familiar hangout spots... one only needs to compare the common behaviour of the earlier months (those of the first lockdown) with those from the autumn to notice the obvious differences.

Between March and June everyone found themselves stuck wherever they were and, whereas many fell prey to despair, many others have been driven to 'work' individually or as part of a group, resorting to defensive and protective rituals that followed a similar pattern.

Space became a starting point: cleaning the house, planning out days, taking care of groceries. Thus, all houses, big or small, became spaces of the mind. Subsequently, people started opening closets, digging through basements or climbing up in attics just to poke around. They started working with time, thinking over and reworking the past: photographs, videos, garments, clothes, memories... all these 'relics' of bygone days were rediscovered and socialised. Old toys restored. Everything was used to mark the time of stillness. It allowed people to weave narratives, elaborate thoughts, re-open or heal wounds.

Times of introspection, regression, or revision were created.

The familiar 'games' that we summed-up and the related rituals helped many emerge 'unscathed' from the first lockdown, but they could not go on forever. And when reclusion came around again, from October onwards, they turned out to be ineffective. And not only because they had already been tried and explored — experiences already 'consumed' and discarded in the delusion that "everything will be alright", including the attempt to discard and revise them from June onwards; but especially because that nightmare was back. Stronger and more powerful than ever.

In the context of rituals, the failure to embrace — both in the first and the second lockdown — traditional forms of either official or popular religious rites should be noted: San Gennaro was not disturbed, not even online. On the other hand, a new sort of secular faith in 'healthcare' has been found through the acknowledgment and celebration of the essential work of doctors and nurses, whose importance is now being reclaimed by treating them as heroes and going as far as establishing a remembrance day for them. Of course, all of this counterbalances the fact that:

> If today we are experiencing a shortage of doctors, hospitals, and beds, it is because of budget cuts: public financing was reduced, small hospitals were shut down, healthcare professionals were downsized, and colossal private medical groups were propelled.[5]

But amid the general, widespread, and globalised crisis — and supported by the tyranny of emergency — no one dwelled on analyzing this data, or examining the causes or verifying why the virus' warning signals had been disregarded,[6] and not even why societies have not been able to appropriately welcome an "unexpected yet not new main character".[7]

From New York City's World Trade Center deaths, to the thousands of missing people in the Mediterranean Sea, to Covid's death toll, the new century seems to be characterised by many occasions where people have experienced a lack of rituals — an observation that brought Adriano Favole to coin the expression "*riti impossibili*" ("impossible rituals").[8] And if in the earlier months of the pandemic, as I have mentioned before, there had been several attempts at reframing, rethinking, and reimagining rituals, at the end of 2020 the social background had completely changed: if at first distress prevailed — accompanied by the eagerness to overcome a moment that, 'they said' would have been brief — from an ethnographic

---

5   Adriano Prosperi, *Un tempo senza storia. La distruzione del passato* (Turin: Einaudi, 2021), p. 120.
6   David Quammen, 'The Warnings. Why we should have known to prepare for COVID-19', The New Yorker, 11 May 2020, pp. 16–22.
7   Prosperi, p. 117.
8   Adriano Favole, 'Confini, socialità, riti', in Aime, Favole, and Remotti, p. 105.

assessment, it emerges that the dominant feelings of the second lockdown were anguish and anxiety.

Accompanied by loneliness.

'We do not know who to turn to', Alberta, a sixty year-old woman from Milan, tells me. Her husband is on *cassa integrazione* (wage guarantee fund) and her children are out of work.

We spend more than we earn. We have reduced our expenses to a minimum. But once the fixed costs are covered, little is left for food. We get by, we take any job available but they are hard to come by. I have cleaned houses myself but since October no one wants me anymore because they are afraid to get infected. This is also a common excuse, people are groping in the dark, no one knows how long this situation will last and they would rather save their money.

During a site–visit at Caritas' soup kitchens in the centre of Milan, I am told that, according to their data, visits have tripled since October. The same had happened a while later at the *mensa del Carmine*, in Naples.

In this second lockdown the hardest and most complicated challenge is financial: 'At first we tried to make do with our reserves. But then? We used up our savings and we do not know what to do'.

With the exception of the wealthy class and people with the most guaranteed jobs, misery is striking everyone. There is no other hope other than mutual support.

3. *Kinds of Solidarity*

A situation such as this led to the rebirth, revival, or increase of some forms of solidarity. But what kinds? The most popular, the institutional one, the one that is publicly recognised, mainly concerns those organisations that put in place and implemented a sort of widespread form of welfare made possible by the involvement and participation of groups of citizens who made themselves available for fundraisers and charity events. All the resources accumulated were then distributed through the reference networks of each association.

Meanwhile a support system made up of micro-activities also took place and expanded: some of these activities relied on religious connections, while others on political participation. For instance, the capillary action of local priests working for those in need. After years in which their public role has been, if not absent, at least very limited, it was as if, through the crisis, they had re-discovered their old role as local authorities and the connected function of social workers acting in their social role as the needle on the scale between those who have more and those who have less. And so, I saw many of them mobilise the circle of most devout and willing worshippers and diligent parishioners to organise food collections and distributions. At the same time it is worth mentioning the significant activity of political groups such as Potere al Popolo, which set up a serious network of support geared towards the most indigent strata in urban areas and hinterland districts where the activists's operating headquarters are located.

In addition to these attempts, some of which were successful, while others less so, there has been a third way, which we must acknowledge as the most important, and perhaps the strongest and most widespread: the resurgence of those forms of solidarity that we could call traditional or 'classic'. In the first place, kin-based networks and parental mutual aid were rekindled, resumed, or started.

If there is one thing that, this year, allowed some very diverse Italian environments to unite and come together again, it was the family. Between October and January, in Milan, Rome and Naples, the three cities that I observed, I noticed that people were building new relationships or rekindling familial bonds that were also working as replacements for public mutual assistance programs or in the absence of state aid. The same happened, as we will see in the coming pages, with completely different modalities, in the context of friendship networks.

A new trend is remote communal dining: people eat together but in different homes; they order take out, they send food packages, they deliver ready meals.

On Saturdays, when Giulio shops at Piazzale Martini's Pam, he buys pantry staples (such as pasta, tomatoes, canned food, bread, eggs) in excess. Once he gets home, he shares the products in excess among his relatives that are most in need. Of course, he is always armed with an excuse to justify the purchase: either reward points, or soon-to-expire meal vouchers… From what I was able to gather, the "restocking" method tends to occur especially when dealing with distant relatives, whereas with closer kins, people tend to offer money: however much is available and however it is possible to distribute it.

Martina and Franca, two Roman sisters, are holding the future of their entire family in their hands. Six brothers and sisters, with a significant amount of grandchildren, most of whom are married, in matrilocality in the surroundings of Nomentana Batteria. Knowing the dire straits in which the most precarious find themselves, they decided to manage a sort of communal piggy bank, merging their own savings with those of the relatives who can contribute. So, every Friday or Saturday they go see their siblings and grandchildren and hand out goods. Alternatively, they visit once a month with larger gifts.

These are but a few concrete examples from the field, but they are the tip of an iceberg that shows the extent of what we were able to rebuild: a precise and clearly defined trail of support and proximity, kept alive by kinship, that cuts through intranational boundaries.

Family still proves to be a strong network that, as we are able to witness, can be infused with and revived by solidarity. Replenished with, renewed, and strengthened by new meaning. We even came across situations in which contemporary interactions and exchanges brought back distant family memories: "just like our grandparents supported each other during WWII..." I heard more than once. The family narratives and its mythologies created a substrate, a framework, and a solid bedrock for today's exchanges, offering up a past, or a story that worked as a driving force and nourished new and more intense relationships. Had it not been for the pandemic, all this processing and remembering the past would not have taken place.

In addition to that, what we have just mentioned is but a possible course of solidarity. We could sum up a few more.

In the research carried out in Campania we observed how the family lineage coexists with and significantly intersects also relationships with neighbours. If during the first lockdown, interactions with neighbours never went beyond the limits of politeness and mutual support, albeit more formally than substantially, during the second lockdown, those first contacts helped build networks that slowly became stronger and more stable, strengthening the opportunities to create more developed, organised, and future oriented types of relationships, with frequent and continuous exchanges — something that is rarely witnessed in a the context of apartment buildings, among neighbours and acquaintances; in short, between people who are not related.

All these forms of solidarity among relatives and close neighbours mainly concern cases analysed within urban areas; while in the province we discovered that the network of mutual support among neighbours covers a wider area.

I have bothered many friends who live in small towns or villages in Campania — in the provinces of Avellino, Caserta, and Benevento — where they were born and raised, or where they are just very popular because they have been local residents for a long time, and they confirmed, told, and showed the existence of this network of relationships built on the basis of space sharing and territorial knowledge and, further, that it covers a wider area precisely because it works within limited areas.

This situation immediately underscores the difference between urban and provincial areas: here, such connections are more 'felt', consistent, and structured, even without the bonds of kinship; whereas in the city, they rely on more circumscribed physical proximity and are heavily reliant on family networks.

4. *What About the Others?*

Over the past few months, because of hampered mobility, I have not been able to carry out thorough examinations. However, I was still able to ascertain that the situation is even more different in the hinterland areas and city outskirts (such as East Naples, or on the 'borders' with Tor Bella Monaca, for example), where processes of social cohesion are more complex and the relationship between locals and foreigners is harsher. In some cases, the problem is also exacerbated by the fact that these areas were often developed without a specific plan, and without social spaces that allow the opportunity to build a relational fabric (spaces devoted to socialisation such as squares, parks, playgrounds for children, as well as cafes, shopping streets, delegating this function to the closest mall), and, thus, without the opportunity to build an accepted and shared system of exchanges. In these areas, local residents themselves are 'subject' to their neighbours, because they have been forced to be in contact with people they consider either strangers or foreigners. Here, the social circuits tighten, relying mostly on networks of kin or old and established friendship, which lead to unhealthy forms of 'solidarity-by-hostility': united against the Other — be it strangers or foreigners.

Obviously, this is an issue especially for the people who do not have family nearby and those who are not integrated in urban, small-town, or suburban social fabrics. And this mainly concerns "the invisibles", to explicitly quote a popular book by Ralph Ellison.[9]

During the months of the second lockdown, it was difficult for me to locate many of my foreign acquaintances who live day-by-day: some rustling up roadside stalls, some selling flowers, other selling trinkets. These people literally disappeared – they got sucked into the maelstrom of

---

9   Ralph W. Ellison, *Invisbile Man* (New York: Random House, 1952).

undocumented immigrants wandering about the city's main train stations or in the city's outskirts, where they survive in extremely precarious circumstances, exposing themselves to the criminal underworld circles. It is clear how these months reinforced a system that widened the gap between those whose lives are safe, and those whose lives are at risk. This gap becomes an abyss between those who are protected, and those who are invisibles. With the 'advantage' that the latter are unseen. And nobody notices.

5. First Diagnosis

Upon a first wide–scale analysis, based on a group of 20–30 year olds — that I either met in person, when possible, or remotely — some, perhaps predictable, problems emerge: first of all, the question of loneliness. Being stuck at home often leads to consuming or using up all possible commitments and, thus, leaves room for the dilemma of what to do with one's own time: study time becomes endless; direct relationships become impossible unless through digital media. Even the ability to invent new forms of relationality dries up more and more: once the Skype group meeting, the Zoom happy hour, the Facebook live dinner, and FaceTime conversations have been experimented with, the vapidness of these media emerge and they start to feel like empty surrogates of face-to-face meetings. Interpersonal relationships dwindle.

So, if the first lockdown had been characterised by an intense use of technology, where Skype happy hours and video-calls were all the rage, the second lockdown veered toward relational minimalism. An Italian author writes on her Facebook page that "During these days when we cannot see each other, I have a penchant for old-timey phone calls, long conversations with the camera off, without emojis. Without the impression of impossible physical closeness. The intensity of voices and the strength of moments of silence, instead. That is what brings us closer". She writes this in mid–november, in the first year of Covid, when lockdown measures had been resumed for about a month.

All of this is intensified by the complete nullification of the body, an issue that concerns women as much as men. What emerges, then, is a silent world, lived in isolation, afflicted by a complete lack of physical expression which has, in many cases, led to the annihilation of desire.

Of course, this information is incomplete: the direct and immediate data is drawn from an inquiry on around 150 people selected from several places throughout Italy. A sample which may have a limited scope and should be not only expanded, but also crossed, for instance, with 'Covid emergency desks', phone lines made available in many cities to provide psychological support. The number of users, their age, and their requests remain undisclosed, so far. At the same time, femicide cases should be studied thoroughly, and a detailed analysis of family violence should be carried out since the number of cases appears to have significantly increased.

6. *Elders and Youths*

In the climate we are describing, we must highlight two opposite ends of the thread that holds together the scenario that emerged over the past year: elders and youths.

Unfortunately, SARS-CoV-2 mainly affected the elderly population, killing thousands of them. It decimated grandparents and, often, parents. It wiped the slate of family stories clean and chopped off the highest end of the generational ladder on which much was still relying. They were the storytellers of family narratives, the bearers of collective memories, grandparents commonly acting as nannies, or who just financially supported their children, and grandchildren as well. They flew off. Without a trace. Rather, they made room for the world of the 'in-between' and younger generations.

The 40–50 year olds, represented by this 'in-between' keep trying to find a proper and new social and cultural placement, and when they do, it is only with struggle and distress.[10] None of this applies to younger generations.

In recent history and in our near past, when western capitalist societies reached a significant level of general crisis, perceivable on multiple levels of social life — economic, productive, demographic — they would resort to what we could interpret as a cynical release valve: war. A trench warfare in WWI, aerial warfare in WWII. After the latter, and after the introduction of the atomic bomb, wars became unviable, there is a risk of squandering everything that has been won and, in a certain sense, losing the golden goose, since everything can be threatened by total annihilation. In fact, the major powers only allow relatively minor conflicts to happen, or they limit

---

10   On these topics, see my book *Le false libertà. Verso la postglobalizzazione* (Milan: Meltemi, 2017).

themselves to unscrupulously instigate conflicts that might favour their economic interests.

The last century was also the century of young people who, unfortunately, have also been sacrificed in the name of development and progress, to the point that in both wars the death toll for 16 to 28 year olds was extremely high.[11] The new century, however, 'conspired' against them, and put them in a corner.[12] And to add insult to injury they were humiliated, nicknamed '*bamboccioni*' (*big babies*) or 'choosy', just to find themselves deprived of any prospect, because of the pandemic, stuck on a laptop, victims of technology more than ever, and forced to the online consumer market.

Thus, an entire younger universe, which was already marginalised and paralysed, is subject to a type of impotence that only finds redemption in moments that could be defined as 'explosive'. At the end of 2020, in Rome's Pincio neighbourhood, we witnessed clashes between groups of young people who would meet almost exclusively to pick fights. The same happened in Venice, in Gallarate, in Umbria, and it still goes on in more subterranean forms. The lack of coverage around these events almost seems intended. But news travels and, even though there might be multiple reasons behind them (such as gangs settling old scores, or confrontations triggered by romantic rejections or disputes...), they all produce similar results: take over the streets, show off, and exhibit one's own anger and rage, even though all of this only takes on destructive forms, towards themselves and others.

As Ernesto De Martino wrote about 60 years ago, they are 'furious teenagers' moved by 'fear of loneliness', who make room for 'explosions of aggressiveness, without premeditation nor planning, without rhyme nor reason'. They are supported by a self-destructive frenzy that follows 'an urge to destroy', exhibiting their 'power of subversion'. It is the loneliness of fear that is embodied in 'pure destructive fury'.[13]

Situations as extreme as the one we are living, when left unmanaged, may lead to the inhuman. The lack of rules, the absence of rituals and perspectives, the lack of outlook on and expectations for the future — all of this leads to a loss of control and to the explosion of violence leading

---

11   On these topics it is important to acknowledge the interpretation on a wide sociologic landscape given by Goffredo Fofi, *Il secolo dei giovani e il mito di James Dean* (Milan: La nave di Teseo, 2020).

12   Stefano Laffi, *La congiura contro i giovani. Crisi degli adulti e riscatto delle nuove generazioni* (Milan: Feltrinelli, 2014).

13   Ernesto de Martino, *Furore, Simbolo, Valore* (Milan: Il Saggiatore, 2013), pp. 183–84.

our world towards unexplored paths and that might push some down a wayward path to darkness and chaos.

7. Conclusions: A Dry-Run for Extreme Capitalism?

> Predictability can only be combined with responsibility, care, a different and sacred relationship with creation, nature, prevention, attention, tension for the world in which we live. Unpredictability – which is often the outcome of rhetoric, mythologies, personal interests – might be an alibi to not do, a pretext to not take responsibility here and now, to always put off to tomorrow, fueling a sense of impending doom […] The future seems unavoidable, it might not happen, and this very risk, this threat, this fear, coupled with ethics and nostalgia for the future, might be our saving grace. Responsibility, caution, wisdom, future-oriented ethics as a way to contain risks and scale down the unpredictable. The future is not what will happen tomorrow. Rather, it is what we decide, think, and do today to build tomorrow.[14]

As it happens in similar cases, the pandemic, as much as it could have been prevented, also allowed several fundamental questions to emerge. I thus believe that we can't agree with Bernard Henri-Lévy when he writes that

> viruses are dumb; they are blind; they are not here to tell us their stories or to relay the stories of humanity's bad shepherds; and consequently there is no 'good use', no 'societal lesson', no 'last judgment' to be expected from a pandemic, nothing to be drawn from it except simple, unemotional observations on the state of a health system (for example) and the fact that we never spend enough, anywhere, for research teams or hospitals.[15]

No, I do not think it is *just* a matter of healthcare, nor *just* a matter of scientific research. This is about questions concerning the environment, preventive care, and, more importantly, the way we program and plan the future. Such questions challenge the way we use the available data to leverage our abilities to 'imagine' ways to build our future.[16]

---

14   Vito Teti, *Prevedere l'imprevedibile. Presente, passato e futuro in tempo di coronavirus* (Rome: Donzelli, 2020), pp. 57–58.

15   Bernard-Henri Lévy, *The Virus in the Age of Madness*, trans. by Steven B. Kennedy (New Haven & London: Yale University Press, 2020), p. 43.

16   "I asked Khan [of the Center for Disease Control and Prevention] about Covid-19. What went so disastrously wrong? Where was the public-health preparedness that he had overseen at the C.D.C.? Why were most countries—and especially the

Furthermore, such a perspective gives us a chance to look at the future with a different outlook: through and towards equality, ecologic mindfulness towards the world surrounding us, a new and greater regard for nature and respect of the environment. Despite everything, this could have been turned into a great opportunity. To think the whole world over. Many warned us: from Walter Benjamin, not only in *Theses on the Philosophy of History*,[17] to Dwight Macdonald, Albert Camus, Paul Goodman, Nicola Chiaromonte... A chance to stop the *Angelus Novus* that has turned into an angel of death. Honestly, though, I do not think we have embarked on the path towards a project for such a non-hegemonic, non-overbearing future.

Epidemics and pandemics are the dull background noises that accompany the historical evolution of our species, they reset its accomplishments, they bring it back to its original condition of precariousness and dependence on nature. We had forgotten all of this. Suddenly, all that which appeared as signs of unlimited progress, in terms of control over nature and boundless – economic, technological, productive – expansion developed into their opposite and contributed to the explosion and transmission platforms of the angel of death. If the 1348 Black Plague's bacillus travelled for a long time on Genoese ships sailed from Kaffa in the fall of 1347, it only took Covid-19 a few hours to travel across the entire world. [...] But other things have happened since then. What we are talking about is the overturning of the very idea of freedom in neoliberalism; of globalisation as global transformation in a market dominated by the greed of multinational corporations that concentrated the world's wealth in the hands of just a few. And we are talking about the little to no globalisation among the people and their States. The pro-European project that arose from the willingness to erase nationalist sentiments and the imperialist drive that led to WWII turned into a selfish and xenophobic continent withdrawing into itself before our very eyes.[18]

The new century, ushered in by the Twin Towers' nightmare, had to face the 2008 crisis which brought entire economies to their knees, and was extremely difficult to leave behind. We were still living through its aftermath when the pandemic hit. With devastating effects, undoubtedly. Maybe we could start speculating about the fact that, somehow, this crisis

---

U.S.—so unready? Was it a lack of scientific information, or a lack of money? 'This is about lack of imagination', he said" (Quammen, p. 17).

17   Walter Benjamin, *On Concept of History*, in Id., *Selected Writings. Vol. 4, 1938-1940*, ed. by Howard Eiland and Michael W. Jennings (Cambridge: Harvard University Press, 2006), pp. 389–400.

18   Prosperi, p. 119. original text in Italian.

helped someone or played in their hands. Surely, it did not get the world back on track, ascribing to it the role of emergency break, which Benjamin thought revolutions might have.[19] It was thoroughly taken advantage of by the extreme fringes of capitalism instead. Let me clarify that I am not claiming that this coronavirus was man-made, that it was the result of a capitalist conspiracy, or, even worse, of a Jewish-banking plot, as an unfortunate theory sadly reiterated recently.[20] Instead, I do argue that, all things considered, given the system and the methods of so called developed countries and their organisation, where the root causes of the pandemic are to be found, the pandemic itself worked in their favour: it paralyzed the whole world, removing every form of social interaction, exchange and gathering, in the complete absence of alternative spaces of freedom, sharing, and conflict; it forced humans in a state of supreme consumers, and promoted this function in such a way that led them to exponentially increase their consumption. This year, entire warehouses full of more or less outdated tech-equipment, gardening tools, household and DIY utensils were emptied, not to mention those containing the vast repertoire concerning the ultimate great passion of advanced society: cooking.

A weird juncture thus materialized: on the one hand, the inability to move, go out, travel, shop… leads to saving and hoarding. Not surprisingly banks are denouncing the inactivity of many bank accounts of the average customer, keeping their capital inoperative. However, if the perception of danger and risk, the uncertainty of tomorrow, and the complete lack of institutional programs to handle the future are stronger than the banks' attempts to persuade to invest, on the other hand, people are led down another path: they are encouraged, spurred, and invited to spend.

So here is how to take financial advantage of COVID-19: a domestic, mostly family-centered world emerged, closed off and isolated; awkward individuals relying on keyboards to complete all kinds of tasks. All this also outlines and defines a multitude of homebound consumers who, thanks to technological improvements, are able to indulge — between online classes, Zoom meetings and meal prepping — in a spot of retail therapy with a simple click. Or they can visit a supermarket's website and order groceries online. Or peek into large online markets just to browse, and maybe they will find the "extraordinary-today-only" offer that will entice further needless purchases. Or maybe the next one will.

---

19   On this topic see Michael Löwy, *La révolution est le frein d'urgence. Essais sur Walter Benjamin* (Paris: Éditions de l'éclat, 2019).
20   Pasquale Bacco, Angelo Giorgianni, *Strage di Stato. Le verità nascoste della Covid-19*, foreword by Nicola Gratteri (Bergamo: Lemma Press, 2021).

At the end of the day, it was a god–send for those businesses that were able to get rid of a large quantity of capitalised production or to multiply sales for online purchases that this year massively boomed everywhere.

Keeping this mindset means asking whether this pandemic could be interpreted as a sort of dry run for what is awaiting the generations to come. It takes on the form of an eerie sci-fi movie: lonely women and men, whose social life has been annihilated, in a reality that is almost completely ruled by technology, under 'accurate' (to say the least) control of the status apparatuses. A world with no way out. Except through purchases.

At the moment, I have yet to come across any alternative: I do not suppose there are counter-information classes aiming to teach us how to put technology at our service and not the opposite. And maybe that is what we should learn from traditional societies.[21]

Those who predicted a pandemic, without being wizards or prophets, also warned against other future dangers: crises generated by other viruses; the imminent ineffectiveness of antibiotics. However, nothing gets done against these threats. Let alone the fact that this crisis will leave us weaker rather than stronger, given the fact that, when it comes to universal changes, from the means of production to global warming, to nature conservation to mindless meat consumption... very little has been and is being done. And I have no reason to believe there is anything in the works.

Thus, it is necessary for us to protect ourselves from the world by isolating and getting separated, choosing more and more advanced technologies to communicate and to keep distance from the world, while still being able to *touch* it.

Provided one has the magic number to access all of this: those of a debit or credit card.

---

21   On these topics, see my essay 'Tecnologie a portata di touch', *Agalma*, 40 (2020), 19–27.

IRINA PODGORNY

DROUGHT IN PARIS HOLY WATER FONTS

In the liturgy of the Catholic Church, God transmits grace through seven sacraments: baptism, confirmation, the Eucharist, penance, the anointing of the sick, priestly ordination, and marriage. These are administered by their intermediaries on Earth; that is, priests and hosts, holy water, oils, wines and chalices, human and non-human agents who, in times of plague, become potential transmitters of another message: the particles of ribonucleic acids.

Those who, neither alive nor dead, in the last two years have managed to confine believing and non-believing humanity, preventing Christians, idolaters, and iconoclasts of baptisms, marriages, Eucharist, confirmations, confessions and anointing, both extreme and precautionary.

This essay aims to reflect on the media of these sacraments, in particular the use of holy water and the instruments for extreme unction in times of fear and disruption, with particular reference to these months marked by the COVID-19 pandemic. Identified as a cause of respiratory diseases, this is a virus with an RNA genome that spread rapidly, compromising the lives and livelihoods of large parts of the population locally and trans-continentally. And although viruses precede us in the world and are an active agent in the co-evolution of eukaryotes, the emergence of COVID-19 confronted us with human despair in the face of the unknown and unpredictable behaviour of the immediate future. As the Argentinian historian Diego Armus says:

> Some epidemics burst, sicken, kill and end in a relatively short period of time. Others seem like marathons against which, during a dense tangle of uncertainties, it is essential to define and adjust priorities, manage resources that are always insufficient, facilitate social, political and cultural convergences of all kinds [...]. And all this with results that are rarely those expected and in the desired timeframe. As human issues — individual and collective —

uncertainties produce discomfort that can range from mild unease to unbridled fear. Learning to live with them is crucial.[1]

Armus emphasises that it is hard to live with uncertainties and to admit the perplexity they generate. It is hard to admit the vulnerability that our ignorance uncovers[2]. But it is also hard to live with the different dimensions and scales on which the virus acts and interacts with us: a non-human scale, where, paraphrasing Richard Dawkins' metaphor,[3] eukaryotic organisms (animals, fungi, and plants) could be understood as mere survival machines for viruses and bacteria that thrive (or not) thanks to the possibility of adapting to them. This is the scale of the rapid and short timescales of virus mutations and at the same time of the very long timescales of evolution, a scale that contrasts sharply with the second one at stake: that is, the lifespan of living organisms, always short, minuscule, at least in evolutionary terms. In the case of our species, this brings us to the scale and awareness of the life of each individual, centered on a short time, just over 100 years: nothing compared to the long times of evolution and the history of the planet. Knowing that viruses have been emerging constantly for billions of years, that they jump between animal species and that they precede us and will outlive us — a certainty that is only a few decades old — does not seem to serve to ward off the uncertainty and fear produced by one's own death or that of others when it results every day in large numbers and terrifying images of overflowing cemeteries.

Among these uncertainties, the conclusions about the infectious stability, mechanisms, and modes of transmission of the new coronavirus evolved several times and resulted in several changes of habits that, in retrospect, were not always justified. Moreover, some behaviour changes survive even when their ineffectiveness has been proven or they are pointless to maintain. The use of latex gloves when going outside, for example, or the mere assumption that the virus was transmitted through doorknobs.

Although there was early talk of aerosol transmission and the need for a human agent to emit it, in March 2020 some work suggested that the virus remained stable on surfaces for up to three days and could therefore maintain its ability to infect. Some microbiologists, including German virologist Christian Drosten, tried to relativise this conclusion, questioning the media's flippancy in replicating this possibility, explaining that the data

1   Diego Armus, 'Elogio de la mascarilla: epidemias, incertidumbres y civilidad sanitaria', in E. Gullo (ed.), *Libro abierto del Futuro* (Buenos Aires: Argentina Futura - Jefatura de Gabinete de Ministros, 2021), 4–12 (p. 5).
2   *Ibid.*
3   Richard Dawkins, *The Selfish Gene* (Cambridge: Cambridge University Press, 1976).

were ambiguous and that papers published in scientific journals should be read in the context of the laboratory. Drosten set out early in the pandemic to examine the scientific data and evaluate it for the public. At that moment, Drosten said, it was very difficult to distinguish what was important in the large amount of scientific literature that was being published, reports that, far from combating it, contributed to uncertainty, especially when the press propagated the reports with an emphasis on the more tabloid aspects.[4]

These were not what later became known as infodemics or fake news, but were rather research papers taken out of context, with weak evidence, but which were a perfect fit for the sales of news and hygiene or protection products. Propaganda helped to keep these sales going in a discursive context where the fear of touching manifested in the successful sales of alcohol gels, disinfectants, and cleaning products, and in the simple act of washing hands with soap and water (which, despite being the cheapest and most effective strategy, was the most readily forgotten).[5]

The accumulation of gestures and gadgets dedicated to preventing us from "touching the virus" proliferated but also generated new habits. Or rather, they revived some very old ones that, paradoxically, come from historical moments prior to the mere visualisation and definition of viruses in their modern sense.

The liturgy of the Catholic Church, in that sense, becomes ideal for analysing this problem thanks to the relatively long (historical, non-evolutionary) record that allows us to observe continuities and reappearances of objects and manners that survive beyond the frameworks that explain diseases. In particular, this essay deals with the fear of holy water from the font, which, contrary to ordinary water mixed with soap, was removed from churches, considered as a probable breeding ground for disease vectors.[6]

---

4 'Coronavirus-Update: Vorsicht vor Vereinfachungen', Podcast with Christian Drosten, Head of the Department of Virology at the Charité Berlin, 16 March 2020 <https://www.ndr.de/nachrichten/info/14-Coronavirus-Update-Vorsicht-vor-Verein fachungen,podcastcoronavirus132.html> (last access: June 25th, 2021).

5 For example, press reports on the mask developed in collaboration with CONICET teams https://atomprotect.mitiendanube.com/, insist on the topic of the survival of the virus on surfaces, an issue that was valid when the patent was announced in 2020, but not in 2021, when commercialisation began. In this sense, appealing to the name of the Consejo Nacional de Investigaciones Científicas (National Council for Scientific Research) is confusing by appealing to arguments that are no longer entirely valid.

6 Holy water and fonts cannot act as a culture medium or as a breeding ground for viruses. The medium is a laboratory technique consisting of a solution containing

1. *Holy Water*

1.1. *Sprinklers*

In 2020, the baptism of a child with a water pistol became famous for a few moments that are now justly forgotten.[7] The event occurred – or rather was photographed – at the end of May 2020 at Saint Marks Catholic Church, Diocese of Nashville, Tennessee. This was allegedly a measure to separate the child from the priest and keep the baptism liturgy inventive and good-humoured. (Fig. 1)

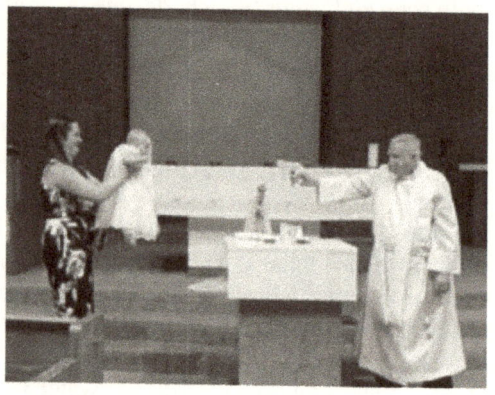

Fig. 1. Fr. Stephen Klasek pretends to shoot water at a baby with a water pistol (source: National Catholic Register, Kettering OH, May 27th, 2020)

---

the necessary nutrients to allow, under favourable conditions, the proliferation of viruses and other agents. Viruses, which are intracellular parasites, need a medium containing living cells, which in principle is not the case with holy water and fonts.

7   Michele La Rosa, 'Holy water and Super Soakers don't mix, priests say', 27 May 2020, <https://catholicherald.co.uk/holy-water-and-super-soakers-dont-mix-priests-say/> (last access: June 25th, 2021).

The Catholic News Agency denied that it was a snapshot of the sacrament. Putting holy water into a squirt gun and treating it as if it were a comedy sketch on SNL is treating both the sacrament and the blessed water unworthily, said Father Pius Pietrzyk, a professor of canon law at St. Patrick's Seminary in California. It was only a joke on the distancing measures then being taken when performing this rite that opens the door to eternal life. The gun, in short, was loaded with ordinary water.

Holy water, in fact, is sacramental, a material object produced by prayers instituted by the Church and intended to sanctify the lives of Catholics, a reference to the purifying power of baptism. Its institution involved a long process in which beliefs about water had to be stripped of the uncleanliness, foulness and muddiness which the devil made credible to the ancient Gentiles about the element of water in the matter of causing purity and cleanliness in souls: the truth being that all was a perpetual filthiness and pitiful pollution in it and even in bodies.[8]

Washing and purifying oneself in the waters of the sea or rivers was a widespread superstition among the ancients, believed in by the modern Moors, the Hindus, and the inhabitants of the West Indies, as well as by Catholics.

Holy water, on the other hand, was water made efficacious by the majesty of the Creator. In the words of Cardinal Juan de Torquemada (1388-1468), "Holy water is water sprinkled with salt, exorcised and sanctified with words of divine prayers, to drive away demons".[9]

Water, before salt is poured into it, signifies human nature, and salt, before it is poured into the water, signifies wisdom or penitence for past faults and caution for future ones. The union of salt and water signifies the hypostatic union of the divine and the human, the bitter conscience that becomes sweetness. Others thought it was the Wisdom and Passion of Christ, or the death of our worms and the spiritual cleansing.

To perform the blessing of holy water, the priest, being in the sacristy where the water and the salt are, dresses himself at dawn and first exorcises the salt with a prayer from the missal, then blesses it and does the same with the water before mixing them and asking that it be for the health of the body and soul of the faithful. He then leaves the sacristy to say high mass, accompanied by the deacon and subdeacon, intones the antiphon *Asperges me Domine*, and sprinkles the altar three times, himself, the deacons, the clergy and finally the people, saying in a low voice, *Miserere mei Deus*.[10]

---

8   José de Santa María, *Triunfo del agua bendita* (Sevilla: Fajardo, 1642), unpaginated.
9   Cited by Santa María, no page.
10   *Ibid.*, no page.

Since the early Middle Ages there has been a liturgical instrument specifically designed for sprinkling holy water: the *aspergilium*, hyssop or aspersorium, used during Easter and other ceremonies. It features a decorated handle with a hollow metal sphere at its end capable of holding the water, which the priest immerses in a container — the holy water vessel — to sprinkle water on the people or things he wishes to bless. (Fig. 2-3)

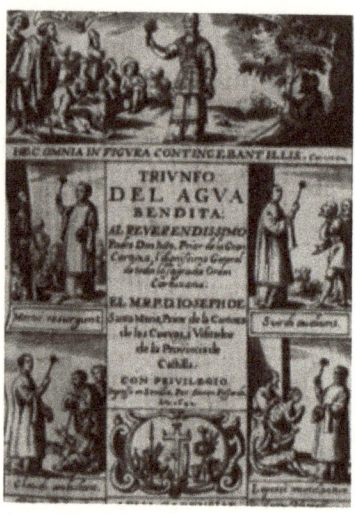

Fig. 2 The use of the sprinkler in *Triunfo del agua bendita*

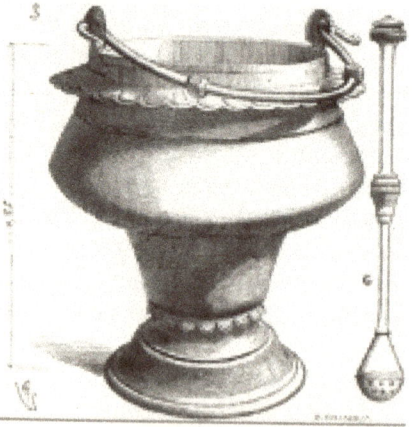

Fig, 3. Holy Water vessel and hyssop

The famous sprinkling water, or holy water, consisted of the ash of the red cow, cedar, the herb hyssop, and of a little scarlet, which, all burnt and turned to ash, were poured into water and served to cleanse and purify the people of the external filth they had contracted for many reasons.[11]

Hyssop thus has a complex genealogy that goes back to pre-Christian times and to medicinal aromatic plants, such as thyme or fennel, to bundles of pig hair and to exorcisms.

But, at the same time, it reminds us that the technology and protocols for administering the sacraments cannot be separated from the first great pandemic wave that went down in history as the Black Death and flared up again and again in different European regions. Museums of sacred art abound in these pieces, showing the importance they had and still have for the sprinkling of water from a distance, even in later times when holy water fonts began to be placed at the entrance to churches.[12]

1.2 *Blessers*

On 29 February 2020, before the World Health Organisation declared a pandemic, Michel Aupetit, the Archbishop of Paris, issued instructions to parish priests on preventing the spread of the coronavirus.[13] These included offering communion only in parishioners' hands and refusing to administer it in the mouth, not offering the chalice to the faithful, asking concelebrants to receive communion by intinction, and not exchanging handshakes as a sign of peace during mass. Likewise, the holy water basins at the entrances of the churches, those that welcome and invite the purification of sins, were to be emptied:

---

11   *Ibid.*, No page.
12   *Ibid.*, No page.
13   It stated: In order to contribute to the fight against this epidemic and to follow the latest recommendations transmitted yesterday evening by M. Michel Aupetit, Archbishop of Paris, has asked all the priests of the parishes of Paris to respect the following measures during Masses and in their church: to offer communion only in the hands of the faithful and refuse to give it in the mouth, not to offer communion in the chalice for the faithful, to ask concelebrants to receive communion by intinction, to ask the faithful not to exchange handshakes as a sign of peace during Masses, to empty the holy water fonts present in the church <https://www.paris.catholique.fr/communique-du-diocese-de-paris-53342.html> (last access: June 25th, 2021).

The first object that comes into view on entering the Church is the holy water font, a vessel designed to contain holy water. The font has its own language: it says to the Christian: "Purify yourselves, you are entering a holy place". This is so much the feeling that the Church wants to inspire that, on the basin of several ancient fountains, this inscription was often engraved: "Wash your sins and not only your face". The use of holy water goes back to apostolic times and the formula for the blessing is attributed to St. Matthew, at least in substance. Every year, on the eve of Easter and Pentecost, the priest blesses a considerable quantity of water, and the faithful do not fail to stock up on it in order to use it advantageously. This is because holy water is sacramental. By virtue of the prayers of the Church and the dispositions of those who use it, holy water remits venial sins for which there is contrition at the time of its use. To obtain this insignificant favour, the physical contact of the water is not necessary, the moral contact is sufficient. The moral contact is made by all the faithful, who, at the moment of the sprinkling which precedes High Mass, testify by a bow of the head that they accept it, although in reality the water does not fall on all of them. Every Christian should have holy water in his house. He must use it often, before prayer, when he gets up and goes to bed; he must especially make it available to the priest when he is called to bring Holy Communion or to give the last Sacraments to a sick person.[14]

And so, at the suggestion of the archbishop, holy water was removed from the church, was no longer offered at the entrance, lost its ability to purify sins, and in fact could become a vehicle for illness and death.

A week later, 'Bénitiers vidés' (*empty blessing fonts*) announced the news, publishing photos of the giant clams (*Tridacna gigas*) that welcome parishioners in many of the country's churches, now without water. Since then, they have remained dry and, in their place, some of them propose to rinse their hands with a ration of alcohol gel, thanks to a bottle installed next to or at the feet of the large mollusk. (Fig. 4)

A similar situation was repeated in León and in different parts of Spain, where, as part of similar measures, it was also proposed that they stop touching or kissing the saints' icons, a custom that does not seem to exist in France, or at least was not regulated there.[15] Thus, each archbishopric, according to the habits of its country, dictated new measures adapted to local customs and rites. This contrasts with the certain universality of furniture and objects destined, for example, to contain and distribute holy water,

---

14   Le Bénitier, *Bulletin paroissial de Saint-Cloud* (19 April 1914), p. 4.
15   <https://www.leonoticias.com/leon/temor-coronavirus-quita-agua-bendita-20200306133352-nt.html> (last access: June 25th, 2021).

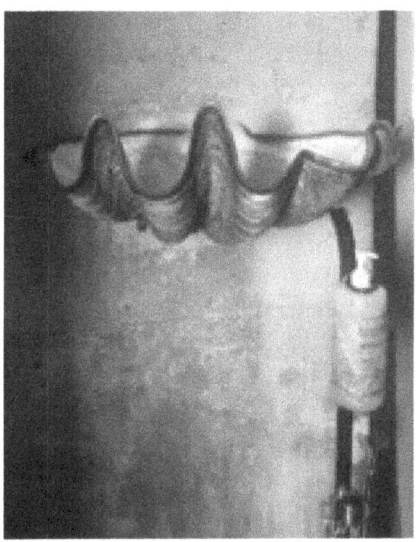

Fig. 4. Holy water font (*bénitier*) from the Saint-Laurent Church in Paris
(Photo by the author)

which are part of a thriving industry that consolidates models and spreads them among the faithful according to fashions and available materials.[16]

The empty holy water fonts shown in European newspapers as a symbol of the pandemic are no longer produced or sold through these channels, but their profusion reveals that they were part of a consumption horizon in Spain and France as well as in Italy, where they can also be found in the churches of San Carlo al Corso in Milan and in the parish church of San Nicola di Bari, in Colonna, near Rome. There, it also gives its name to a literary prize: La Tridacna. However, the drought of the historical tridacnas does not seem to be a novelty: there are testimonies — tourist postcards and photographs of visitors — that show them without water in non-pandemic times. The newspaper headlines and the photo of the dried-up clam can be related, on the other hand, to its natural monumentality, to that presence loaded with symbols where the culture of curiosity, the gratitude of the

---

16　See for example the objects and objectives of the Vaticanum shop, which delivers its products all over the world: <https://www.vaticanum.com/es/benditeras?pagenumber=5&pagesize=30&orderby=0#/specFilters=4m!#-!1048> (last access: June 25th, 2021).

faithful, the fashion for collecting mollusks, and the European colonial or commercial expansion in the oceans of Asia and Africa, as well as the space of the Church as the repository for the greatness of God, are all combined.

Although a history of these objects and their donors has yet to be compiled, heritage inventories in Spain and France show that they have existed as an architectural element in churches since the end of the eighteenth century and that they proliferated especially in the nineteenth century. They are specimens of the subfamily *Tridacninae* and of the giant clam genera *Hippopus* and *Tridacna*, a hermaphroditic bivalve mollusk inhabiting the Red Sea and the Indian and Pacific Oceans, which have been traded and exploited in the past but also in the present. The name *Tridacna* is apparently due to Pliny, and some specimens or their images were known in Rome since antiquity.[17] There are archaeological and ethnographic records of the use of its shell for the manufacture of objects at local or regional level, but the giant clam, whose meat is sold as an exotic delicacy, has been over-collected on a large scale for the food market[18], for aquaria, and, as the visit to the churches shows, as a sacred-liturgical object that connects even the most distant geographies and gives evidence of this traffic in churches both in the capitals and in the provinces. The pandemic, in this way, could help us to conceive a new research project exploring the supply networks of ecclesiastical tridacnas, a 'nomadic object', in the sense suggested by Mia Mochizuki[19]: one more of those earthly objects (marine, in this case) that are integrated into the world of religion. Perhaps it was a fashion imposed from Paris with which more than one devotee wanted to decorate his village church. The truth is that very little is known about the ecclesiastical tridacnas, partly because of the invisibility with which monuments are covered and of which Robert Musil and Andreas Huyssen spoke. Nevertheless, there they are: they continue to welcome the faithful, one half on the right and the other half on the left.

Acquasantiera in Italian, *bénitier* in French, or *benditera* in Spanish: these are the names given to the substance that the tridacna holds but which,

---

17 Although bivalve shells were undoubtedly used as a symbol of female fertility, the giant clams — where the faithful stuck their fingers — should not be confused with the scallops of the scallop family, which is the symbol of St. James and the shell depicted, in exaggerated size, in Botticelli's Birth of Venus.

18 G. Remoissenet, C. Wabnitz, N. Grand-Pittman, V. Sachet & L. Yan, *Guide de collectage de bénitiers* (Communauté du Pacifique, 2015).

19 Mia Mochizuki, 'Connected Worlds. The World, the Worldly, and the Otherworldly: an introduction', in *The Nomadic Object: The Challenge of World for Early Modern Religious Art* ed. by Christine Göttler & Mia Mochizuki (Leiden: Brill, 2018), pp. 1–34.

in the case of the French name, is also used to refer to the clam itself, proving its long history of association and diffusion as an ecclesiastical element. In a 1903 article on the use of snails in zoological industries, the author noted:

> A thousand objects of use are fashioned from the shells. The tridacnas, large bivalves from the Indian Ocean, are used as fonts. In the church of Saint-Sulpice, in Paris, you can see two fonts given to François I by the Republic of Venice.[20]

In other words, they were given as gifts in the sixteenth century — probably for a royal collection — and in the eighteenth century they were mounted on marble pedestals carved by the sculptor Jean-Baptiste Pigalle, who decorated them with octopuses, algae, corals and other zoophytes (Fig. 5).

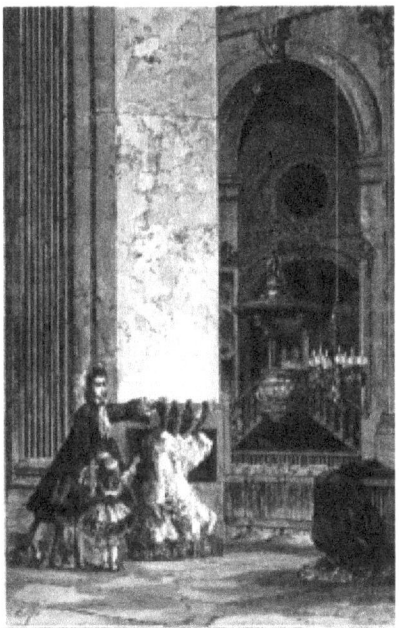

Fig. 5. *Gigantic tridacne*, used as a font in the church of Saint-Sulpice in Paris, taken from Louis Figuier, *La vie et les moeurs des animaux. Zoophytes et mollusques* (Paris: Hachette, 1866), p. 339.

---

20   V. Delosière, 'Les usages des coquilles', *La science illustrée. Recueil encyclopédique* (1903), 107–08 (p. 108).

Another beautiful composition is found in Le Havre, where the mollusk was integrated into an older base with a sculpted eagle.[21] Most of them, on the other hand, are embedded as shelves on the entrance columns, and the material used is different from that of the original construction.

This distance of two hundred years between the gift and the sculpture speaks of a history that the Malacological Museum of Cupra Marittima (province of Ascoli Piceno in the Marche region) recovered in an exhibition in June 2018: 250 objects from all over Europe, dating from the seventeenth century to the present day. According to Tiziano Cossignani, director of the museum, the first holy water fonts were shells. They appeared in churches in the seventeenth century as a handcrafted product stylised in stone or other materials, while the use of the shells in churches across France dates from the following century. In Germany, on the other hand, holy water fonts were fashioned in porcelain, while in Italy all ceramic production sites have produced and continue to produce shell-shaped holy water fonts.

Today, thanks to their supposed casting, we can see them in all their splendour, with the edges finished in bronze, as in the case of the French ones, or in ebony wood with mother-of-pearl inlays, like the half-preserved shell in Zaragoza, which is thought to have arrived from the Philippines on the occasion of the 1908 Spanish-French Exhibition held to commemorate the first centenary of the Sieges of Zaragoza.[22] A reminder of the end of a war and of the city's role in upholding the glory of Spain, it is kept in a school museum.

2. *Social distance and sacraments in times of plague*

Several historians have noted the crises triggered by successive waves of plague in Europe. From the first wave in the fourteenth century, the Church emerged richer but also more battered: it had not found an answer to the question of why God had imposed such a trial on humanity, nor had it provided spiritual assistance when it was needed.

Ugo Buoncompagni (1502-1585), Pope Gregory XIII, ordered the bishops, in accordance with the Council of Trent— where he had acted as adviser to the papal legate — to proceed against parish priests who did not maintain their residence in time of plague. As for the obligation to

---

21   <https://gallica.bnf.fr/ark:/12148/btv1b105865154.r=b%C3%A9nitier?rk= 429186;4> (last access: June 25th, 2021).

22   <http://ceres.mcu.es/pages/Viewer?accion=4&AMuseo=IESGZ&Ninv=G0822> (last access: June 25th, 2021).

administer the Eucharist to the plague victims, theologians were sharply divided. Some proposed to leave the host on a table in the sick person's house in a corporal, on a small plate or on the paten, so that he could take it on his own, but this required the permission of the diocesan bishop.

The doctors of Salamanca and many others held, however, that there was no obligation: this sacrament was not so necessary as to sacrifice for a dying person. This opinion seems to follow Buoncompagni's statement addressed to his former pupil, Cardinal Carlo Borromeo, Archbishop of Milan, who had asked him whether the sacraments were administered in times of plague. The answer came on 12 October 1576, at the height of the Milanese plague, which had occurred during his episcopate, due in part to the great influx of the faithful to Milan, a city for which he had obtained the extension of the Roman Jubilee of the previous year. But the Milanese jubilee was to last only a few weeks. On 17 April, the governor, concerned about the cases of plague in Venice and Mantua, limited pilgrimages to the city, only to ban them definitively in July, when the first episodes were recorded in the city. On 11 August, the plague was proclaimed, and the governor abandoned the city for a safer place. The archbishop, then in Lodi, returned immediately and, with militant Christianity, devoted himself to bringing relief to the sick. Barefoot, holding the relic of the holy nail inserted in a wooden cross built for the occasion, he marched in procession to ask for the extinction of the plague. He ordered that only adults should accompany him, in single file and at a distance of three metres from each other. Borromeo is today the patron saint of Lombardy and is invoked against ulcers, intestinal disorders, and stomach diseases. The plague had disappeared in 1578, giving him time to demonstrate his devotion.

The risk for priests, needless to say, increased with extreme unction, a sacrament in which no mucous membrane was left untouched because it is performed in two ways: one proximate and one remote. The remote is the oil (which had to be olive oil) blessed by the bishop, and the proximate is the anointing, which the priest does with his fingers in the form of a cross and on the organs of the five senses, the first locations of man's disconcerts and sins. The kidneys and feet were also anointed, although for the sake of honesty, those of women were left out. Faced with a normal dying man, after the anointing in the form of a cross, the priest had to wipe his hands with breadcrumbs or bran, and wash and dry them. The rags, bread, and water were thrown into the fire and the ashes into the pool. In times of plague, on the other hand, anointing could be done by means of a long wand which was burnt after use or kept for the next eviction after careful cleaning. (Fig. 6)

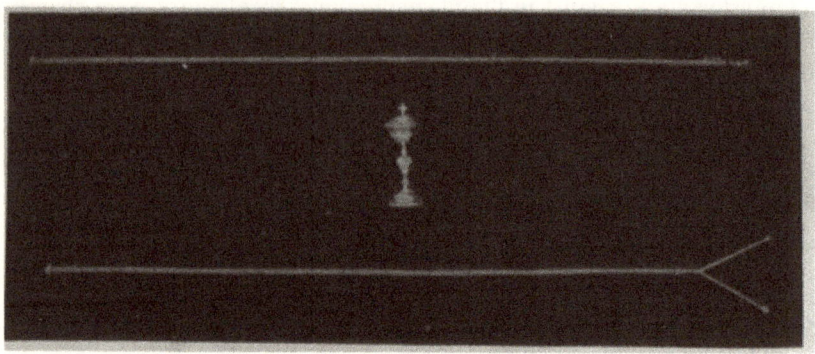

Fig. 6. Rod for Holy Communion and pitchfork for the
Extreme Unction of the plague victims, 17th century.

Let us not forget that in those years, the practice of isolating the sick
and avoiding touching them to prevent contagion was consolidated and
systematised. The idea of quarantine took on biblical significance; the
Flood and other events referred to in the holy books would have lasted
forty days, a metaphorical figure which, as can be seen in the quarantine
provisions enforced in Europe today, can last from 7 to 14 days, sometimes
11 or 10. In China, on the other hand, it lasts 28.

3. *Conclusions*

Fear and uncertainty are not sterile: they produce realities, generate
new objects, recycle or make old ones visible, revive beliefs buried by
history. They are transformed into measures which change from country
to country and which are expressed, for example, in the obligatory or
non-obligatory wearing of masks outdoors, being able to carry out
physical activity in public spaces, the number of days quarantines are
made up of. These differences show the fragmentation of opinions in the
world of health advisors at the national level, but also demonstrate how
living with the fears caused by the pandemic is modelled on different
local scales.

On the other hand, the behaviour and evolution of the virus reinforce
several elements that, for several decades, have accompanied us as

theoretical themes in the history and philosophy of science, in particular in the history of the investigation of epistemic things and scientific objects. I am referring to their emergence and possible disappearance, to the role of unexpected events in the possibility of observing or conceptualising the previously unseen and, in that sense, of the place of the unpredictable or the predicted in the production of new knowledge[23].

This and any other virus, or pandemic, create an ideal situation to "observe" in real time the mechanisms of organic and inorganic evolution, a mute, permanent presence that occurs beyond human will and that, for various reasons, is excluded from our perception of what constitutes our everyday life. No one, since the end of the nineteenth century, can ignore it, nor that bacteria and viruses are part of this system of life on earth that contains us and determines us as a species. The pandemic, we might say, catches us unawares because we do not, after all, take our animal nature seriously, nor do we understand its consequences beyond the world of ideas. Being a eukaryote is much more than an identity label.

Lorraine Daston and Peter Galison argued that the rapidity of change in the sciences in the late nineteenth and early twentieth centuries shaped the critique of objectivity.[24] In this third decade of the twenty-first century, the accelerating change of things (in this case, of a nucleic acid particle) has crept into everyone's lives (whether at the level of virus mutations, vaccine production or changing research results). It is impossible to foresee where it might lead us. And that — as Klaus Wowereit, former mayor of Berlin, said — is good.

Acknowledgements

I am grateful to the colloquium organisers Corinna Guerra and Marco Piazza for the invitation to participate in this volume as well as for their comments and patience. To them I must add the names of Juan José Morrone, Antonio Eusebio Lazcano Araujo Reyes, Esteban Buch, Maribel Martínez Navarrete, Nathalie Richard and Susana García who

---

23 Cf. Lorraine Daston (ed.), *Biographies of Scientific Objects* (Chicago: University of Chicago Press, 2000); Hans-Jörg Rheinberger, *Toward a History of Epistemic Things: Synthesizing Proteins in the Test Tube* (Stanford, California: Stanford University Press, 1997).
24 Lorraine Daston, Peter Galison, *Objectivity in historical perspective* (New York: Zone Books, 2007).

made valuable suggestions to early versions of this work which is part of the RISE SciCoMove Project (Scientific Collections on the Move), funded by the European Union through its Horizon 2020 programme for scientific research and innovation and Marie Sklodowska–Curie Grant No. 1011007579.

AUREO LUSTOSA GUERIOS

SOME REASONS FOR THE RE-EMERGENCE OF THE PLAGUE METAPHORS DURING THE CORONAVIRUS PANDEMIC

1. *Remembering the Plague as a pandemic habit*

Since its start, the coronavirus pandemic has conditioned all areas of life, influencing our scientific, political, and economic agendas, as well as our social, cultural, and even religious interactions. Unsurprisingly, the pandemic has dominated media attention, with newspapers, TV channels, and websites reviewing and conjecturing about it from every possible angle. In an effort to understand the crisis, journalists and reporters would often turn to history and examine the experience of previous pandemics. Nevertheless, their discussions customarily passed over health emergencies of the present or near past to focus, instead, on the plague experience of prior centuries. Little thought was given, for instance, to the fact that the COVID-19 pandemic was not the only active pandemic of 2020, but rather the third — the other two being the HIV/AIDS Pandemic, active since the 1980s, and the Seventh Cholera Pandemic, which broke out in 1961 it was never declared over. More recent health crises, such as the 1968 Flu Pandemic (the so-called Hong Kong flu) or even the 1918 Influenza Pandemic (Spanish flu), have also drawn little attention from the media and the public, something which may be quite surprising given that they happened in a world similar to our own and that they share many of the coronavirus features (viral infection, airborne transmission, high morbidity, comparable mortality rates).

The historical outbreaks of bubonic plague, however, were customarily mentioned by the press. A habit was formed of drawing parallels to the health crisis of the fourteenth to the eighteenth centuries, especially in the early months of the pandemic, when the idea of it still seemed novel and abnormal. On the one hand, the choice of the plague as a standard for comparison may seem natural since, among the population, the Black Death is probably the best-known pandemic. Yet, on the other, the choice is also surprising given that the plague occurred in societies that differed enormously from our own, and that its medical aspects do not compare to COVID-19 very well — their mortality rates are unrelatable, for example. This chapter seeks to explore some of the intricacies of the cultural responses to the plague and the coronavirus.

2. *A brief history of the Plague*

The plague is a bacterial infection caused by *Yersinia pestis*, which is usually disseminated by the bite of fleas, especially those of rodents. After lodging in the flea's gut, the bacterium produces a biofilm that blocks its digestive tract and, consequently, impedes digestion. As a result, the starved flea searches desperately for hosts, trying to drink their blood just to regurgitate it moments later alongside *Yersinia pestis*. Although usually blamed solely on rats, the plague's natural reservoir is constituted of rodents in general — which account for about 40% of all mammals — so squirrels, hamsters, marmots, and others, may also spread the disease. Once it spreads among wild animals, the plague may become endemic to an area, with potentially infected populations likely existing today in the USA, Brazil, Madagascar, India, China, Kazakhstan, and elsewhere.[1]

Once inside the human body, *Yersinia pestis* may multiply for a few days, resulting in an incubation period of typically two to six days. After symptoms surface, the infection may develop into three different variants, depending on the mechanism of contagion and events within the victim's body. In its most common form, *bubonic plague*, the pathogen attacks the lymphatic system, causing the lymph nodes to swell into characteristic buboes that may appear in the groin, neck or armpit. The *septicaemic plague* occurs when the pathogen targets the circulatory system, which allows it to reach nearly all parts of the body and causes the blood to coagulate and the patient to bleed internally. Finally, there is *pneumonic plague*, which infects the lungs, compromising the respiratory system and conferring to the pathogen the capacity of spreading directly through the air. All three forms result in fever, headaches, nausea, and weakness. Gangrene may also occur, especially in the extremities (fingers, toes and nose). Difficulty in

---

1   'Global distribution of natural plague foci as of March 2016', World Health Organization, 15 March 2016, online. <https://www.who.int/images/default-source/health-topics/plague/plague-map-2016.png?sfvrsn=68bcc3ee_4> (last access: March 5th, 2021).

breathing is common in the septicaemic and pneumonic forms, as well as coughing and vomiting blood.[2] As with other diseases, plague's mortality rates vary in conformity with a range of factors; yet, if untreated, bubonic plague results in death in 50% to 80% of cases, while the septicaemic and pneumonic forms are almost always fatal. To allow for comparison, smallpox lethality was of about 30%,[3] untreated cholera may get to 60%,[4] while Ebola averages at 50%, although it can reach 90% on occasion.[5] Since plague can be treated with antibiotics, current mortality rates are around 11% if the infection is detected in time.[6] Albeit more bearable, the figure continues to be quite intimidating.

The pathogen was observed for the first time in 1894 by Alexandre Yersin and Kitasato Shibasaburo during an outbreak in Hong Kong. In 1898, Paul-Louis Simond identified the flea as a vector, thus establishing the habitual mechanism of contagion — a crucial piece of information to draw prevention strategies. Since then, historians have long wondered if the Black Death was caused by *Yersinia pestis* or not. Confirmation only came in 2010, when a genetic study using two independent methods attested that individuals found in plague pits located across Europe had actually died of bubonic plague.[7] Then, in 2013, another investigation using samples from a collective burial site in Germany confirmed that the Plague of Justinian in the sixth century was also caused by the plague.[8] Thus, current historians

2   Sandra W. Moss, 'Bubonic Plague', in Joseph P. Byrne, *Encyclopedia of Pestilence, Pandemics, and Plagues* (London: Greenwood Press, 2008), pp. 74–76.

3   Victoria A. Harden, 'Smallpox', in Byrne, p. 647.

4   Donato Gómez-Diaz, 'Cholera: First through Third Pandemics', in Byrne, p. 98.

5   'Ebola virus disease', World Health Organization, 21 June 2020, <https://www. afro.who.int/health-topics/ebola-virus-disease#:~:text=Ebola%20virus%20 disease%20(formerly%20known,rate%20of%20up%20to%2090%25> (last access: March 5th, 2021).

6   'What is plague?', CDC Centers for Disease Control and Prevention, <https:// www.cdc.gov/plague/faq/index.html> (last access: March 5th, 2021).

7   Stephanie Haensch and others, 'Distinct clones of Yersinia pestis caused the black death', *PLOS pathogens*, (October, 7, 2010), <https://doi.org/10.1371/journal. ppat.1001134> (last access: March 5th, 2021).

8   Michaela Harbeck and others, 'Yersinia pestis DNA from Skeletal Remains from the 6th Century AD Reveals Insights into Justinianic Plague', *PLOS Pathogens*, (May 2, 2013), <https://doi.org/10.1371/journal.ppat.1003349> (last access: March 5th, 2021); David M. Wagner and others, 'Yersinia pestis and the Plague of Justinian 541–543 AD: a genomic analysis', *The Lancet Infectious Diseases*, 14, 2014(4), 319–26.

speak of at least three worldwide conflagrations: the *First Plague Pandemic* in Antiquity (541–747), the *Second Plague Pandemic* in the Middle Ages and Modern Period (c. 1330-1844), and the *Third Plague Pandemic*, which began in the nineteenth century and ended in the 1930s[9] or 1960s,[10] or — as some argue —is still ongoing.[11] However, it is important to note that this tripartite scheme might be expanded in the near future. There is evidence that the plague infected humans since at least 3000 *BCE*,[12] with scholars recently arguing that a fourth plague pandemic might have taken place before all others, possibly being responsible for the Neolithic Decline (about 3400 *BCE*).[13]

3. *How plague became the Mother of all Plagues*

The fact that some historians consider the Third Pandemic to be ongoing may sound surprising to some. That is due to a Eurocentric tradition that asserts that the plague 'disappeared' after the Plague of Marseille ended in 1722. Simply put, it did not: there were outbreaks in Central and Eastern Europe in 1738, in Russia in 1770 or in the Ottoman Empire in 1801. Italy experienced a dreadful eruption in Sicily in 1743, which was viewed in terms of continuity by a chronicler at the time: "[The contagion] was little inferior to the one which afflicted the Capital in the year of 1656, because [...] over 43.400 people [...] were calculated extinct in the period of fewer than three months".[14] In fact, Italy would register its last plague outbreak

---

9   Monica H. Green, 'Editor's Introduction to "Pandemic Disease in the Medieval World: Rethinking the Black Death"', in Ead. (ed.), *Pandemic disease in the medieval world: rethinking the black death* (Bradford: Arc Humanities Press, 2015), 9–25 (p. 10).

10   John M. Theilmann, 'Plague in the Contemporary World', in Byrne, pp. 514–16.

11   J. N. Hays, *Epidemics and pandemics: their impacts on human history* (Santa Barbara: Abc-clio, 2005), pp. 331–44.

12   Simon Rasmussen and others, 'Early divergent strains of Yersinia pestis in Eurasia 5,000 years ago', *Cell*, 163.3 (2015), 571–82; Julian Susat and others, 'A 5,000-year-old hunter-gatherer already plagued by Yersinia pestis', *Cell Reports*, 35, 2021(13), 109278.

13   Nicolás Rascovan and others, Emergence and Spread of Basal Lineages of Yersinia pestis during the Neolithic Decline, *Cell*, 176, 2019(1-2), 295–305.

14   "Poco respettivamente [il contagio] fu inferiore a quello, che afflisse questa Capitale nell'anno 1656, perché [...] più di 43400 persone [...] computaronsi estinte fra lo spazio di meno di tre mesi". My translation. Orazio Turriano, *Memoria istorica del contagio della città di Messina dell'anno 1743* (Naples: Domenico Terres, 1745), preface, no page number provided. Available at: <http://

only in 1815, in the area around Bari. That happened just two decades before the country was ravaged by a novel affliction: cholera.

Therefore, the Plague of Marseille of 1720 does not mark the end of the plague in Europe nor the World. If we widen our gaze to include broader geopolitical areas — after all, pandemics are continent-wide by definition — this celebrated checkpoint reveals itself to be illusory and arbitrary.[15] Even during the twentieth century, there were relevant eruptions in industrialised countries, as proven by the outbreaks of Porto in 1898 or Glasgow, Sidney, and San Francisco in 1900. As it happens, the USA has had at least 1,006 confirmed and probable plague cases between 1900 and 2012; sixteen cases and four deaths occurred as recently as 2015.[16] Moreover, in late 2017, an outbreak happened in Madagascar, resulting in a total of 2,417 cases and 209 deaths (8.6% mortality).[17] To be sure, these eruptions were small in scale and did not reach the enormous mortality rates of previous centuries; but still, they took place. If they were not successfully managed, they could have just as well gotten out of control.

Current events have shown us that epidemics do not inevitably bow before human will. As Monica Green convincingly argues, recent experiences with SARS, Ebola and now COVID-19 urge new plague surveys to rethink the Black Death on a global scale, abandoning the exaggerated emphasis on Europe.[18]

This "disappearance narrative" overlooks the plague's nature as a pandemic and, therefore, does not make justice to the planetary scale of the phenomenon. The scholarship has traditionally concentrated on the European experience of the Middle Ages and Early Modern period to the detriment of more recent experiences which took place elsewhere. The Third Plague Pandemic is often put aside by this version of the story, even if it was in this period that the bacterium was discovered. Mortality rates

www.bibliotecanapoletana.it/archivio/medicina/220> (last access: March 5th, 2021).

15   Green, 'Editor's Introduction to "Pandemic Disease in the Medieval World: Rethinking the Black Death"', p. 14.

16   'Plague in the United States', CDC Centers for Disease Control and Prevention, 25 November 2019, <https://www.cdc.gov/plague/maps/index. html#:~:text=Over%2080%25%20of%20United%20States,in%20people%20 ages%2012%E2%80%9345> (last access: March 5th, 2021).

17   Van Kinh Nguyen and others, 'The 2017 plague outbreak in Madagascar: Data descriptions and epidemic modelling', *Epidemics*, 25 (2018), 20–25.

18   Monica H. Green, 'Taking "Pandemic" Seriously: Making the Black Death Global', in Ead. (ed.), *Pandemic disease in the medieval world: rethinking the black death*, pp. 27–61.

were no less striking at this point: at least ten million individuals lost their lives in India alone.[19]

Several reasons underlie this selective narrative memory. Eurocentrism is certainly a motivator, as are more practical reasons such as the difficulties inherent to interdisciplinary research, language barriers, obstacles to access sources, or simply the lack of appropriate technology — genetic surveys became prevalent only in the past decade or so.

Beyond that, a key reason to sustain the narrative is the terrifying magnitude of the death toll. Historians agree that at least 30% to 40% of the European population perished during the Black Death (1346–1353),[20] with some arguing that numbers could be as high as 60%.[21] If, as many believe, the population of Europe was 75 million in 1346, it probably diminished by 1353 to around 40 to 50 million.[22] Regardless of what the precise numbers might be, this was clearly an event of massive proportions. It constitutes the sole episode in human history in which the global population decreased, resulting in a halt for about a century in the relentless growth of humankind.[23] According to Biraben's calculations, the world's population shrank from 443 million in 1340 to 374 million in 1400 – a net difference of sixty-nine. Only by 1500, it would grow again to 460 million.[24]

Although other afflictions may have reached similar or perhaps higher numbers, they do not come even close to match the plague's proportional distribution within the population (morbidity rate). The AIDS pandemic, for example, has caused the death of an estimated 32.7 million people up to 2019,[25] while smallpox is thought to have put an end to 300 million lives in the twentieth century alone.[26] Yet, their wide distribution in time and space affected society in very distinct ways. The sole exception is the demographic collapse that followed the Colombian exchange in the sixteenth century. It was caused by successive outbreaks of various diseases — above all

---

19   Hays, p. 332.
20   Byrne, p. XXIII.
21   Ole J. Benedictow, *The Black Death, 1346–1353: the complete history* (Woodbridge: Boydell Press, 2004), p. 300.
22   Hays, p. 62.
23   Colin McEvedy and Richard Jones, *Atlas of World Population History* (New York: Facts on File, 1978), pp. 342–51 (p. 346).
24   Jean Noël Biraben, 'An essay concerning mankind's demographic evolution', *Journal of Human Evolution*, 9.8 (1980), 655–63 (table 2, p. 658).
25   'Global HIV & AIDS statistics — 2020 fact sheet', UNAIDS, <https://www.unaids.org/en/resources/fact-sheet> (last access: March 5th, 2021).
26   Donald A. Henderson, 'The eradication of smallpox – an overview of the past, present, and future', *Vaccine*, 29 (2011), D7–D9 (p. D8).

smallpox — which decimated the New World's autochthonous populations. However, the enormous loss of life was accompanied by other phenomena which attracted more cultural interest at the time and, in general terms, the misplaced attention worked to silence this experience and erase it from collective memory. So much so that only after the 1970s historians have revaluated the demographic collapse following the Columbian exchange as a crucial axis in the interaction between the Old World and the New.[27] A comparable argument can be made for the Influenza Pandemic of 1918. Despite its enormous death toll, variously estimated at between 50 and 120 million, the pandemic's partial overlap with the First World War distracted cultural attention enough for it to be declared forgotten by historians.[28]

In this way, the Second Plague Pandemic turns out to be unique on the scale of its impact. It has left profound marks in politics, economics, culture and even religion. Indeed, its cultural imprint is so significant that the plague was transformed into the disease *par excellence*, often in overlap with the ideas of Death or Apocalypse itself. That happened for a variety of reasons, chief among which is the calamitous mortality it inflicted, and the repercussions connected to that event.

Beyond that, there is the cyclical nature of the plague outbreaks, which would not fade after a few years but would rather run their course periodically every generation or so. Biraben estimates that there was at least one localised plague outbreak in Europe every year between 1347 and 1670.[29] In the sixteenth century alone, there were five extensive eruptions in 1400, 1438–1439, 1456–1457, 1464–1466, and 1481–1485.[30] William Shakespeare was born shortly before an outbreak in 1564 and would encounter the disease five more times before his death in 1616. This recurrent pattern ensured that the plague could not be ignored or forgotten. For at least five centuries, its threat was too real and present to be put aside, something which resulted in profound collective fears and anxieties. In that sense, the trauma inflicted by the plague is crucially different from that caused by other similar events. The Influenza Pandemic of 1918, for example, lasted for slightly less than two years and seemingly vanquished

---

27   Alfred W. Crosby, *The Columbian exchange: biological and cultural consequences of 1492* (Santa Barbara: Greenwood Publishing Group, 2003); Crosby, *Ecological imperialism: the biological expansion of Europe, 900-1900* (Cambridge: Cambridge University Press, 2004).

28   Alfred W. Crosby, *Americas forgotten pandemic: the influenza of 1918* (Cambridge: Cambridge University Press, 2003).

29   Hays, p. 46.

30   *Ibid.*

afterwards, allowing for its collective memory to abate and quietly blend with the cultural shock caused by the First World War. The plague, however, would not go away; its shadow would loom large as an enduring menace for generations. This cyclical nature favoured the emergence of personal and collective habits designed to cope with the crisis, control the spread of disease, and relieve psychological stress. The memory of the plague would not be obfuscated by other social or cultural phenomena.

Moreover, since nearly all contagious diseases tended to be interpreted as 'plagues', the *idea of plague* would be carried on by other diseases after plague outbreaks became smaller and less frequent in Europe. Between 1830 and 1900, the continent was hit by four momentous Cholera Pandemics, which affected society in many ways but without ever approaching the enormous relevance of the Black Death. That notwithstanding, people would frequently interpret the two diseases as one and the same: it was common for writers, chroniclers, and physicians at the time to call cholera 'the plague'. Alexander Pushkin, for example, wrote *A Feast in Time of Plague* (1830) while in isolation due to the Cholera Quarantine of Moscow. In 1771, the city had experienced a severe plague outbreak, so its first encounter with cholera sixty years later — well within living memory — was naturally interpreted by most as a re-enactment of a past experience. Similarly, when cholera emerges in Eugène Sue's best-selling popular novel *The Wandering Jew* (*Le Juif Errant*, 1844), it is accompanied by an author's footnote:

> In 1346, the famous black plague devastated the globe; its symptoms were the same as cholera, and the same inexplicable phenomenon of its gradual progress in stages and along a given route. In 1660 another similar epidemic decimated the world again.[31]

The plague outbreaks of 1346 and 1660 are seen here as the direct predecessors of the cholera outbreak of 1832. The epidemics might have distinct names, yet, in practice, their supposedly shared symptoms and transmission patterns turn them into one and the same.

---

31   "En 1346, la fameuse peste noire ravagea le globe ; elle offrait les mêmes symptômes que le choléra, et le même phénomène inexplicable de sa marche progressive et par étapes selon une route donnée. En 1660 une autre épidémie analogue décima encore le monde". Eugène Sue, *Le Juif errant* (Bruxelles: Méline, Cans et compagnie, 1844), vols 7–8, part XIII, chapter X, p. 145; my translation.

Curiously, the confusion could also happen the other way around. In *The Innocents Abroad* (1869), Mark Twain claims to witness in Venice a grand fete honouring a saint who had been instrumental in doing away with cholera three hundred years before.[32] Rather, the *Festa di San Rocco* is dedicated to the plague-deliverer Saint Roch, and is celebrated annually since 1576 to commemorate the end of an acute plague outbreak. Twain is confusing the eruptions of cholera and plague — and probably on purpose.

The cultural confusion with plague also extends to other transmissible diseases, a strategy that allowed artists to enrich discourses on any affliction by using plague metaphors. In literature especially, almost any malady can be transformed into plague: Jack London's *The Plague Ship* (1897) is actually about yellow fever; *The Plague* (*A Peste*, 1910) by Brazilian author João do Rio portrays smallpox; Gesualdo Bufalino's *The Plague Sower* (*La Diceria dell'Untore*, 1981) is built upon tuberculosis; while the popular sci-fi novel *Journals of the Plague Years* (1988) by Norman Spinrad is an early discussion of AIDS.

Furthermore, these links and exchanges do not rely solely on culture but are frequently also based on outdated science. Until the rise and acceptance of the *Germ Theory of Disease* from the 1860s onwards, most diseases were seen as ultimately caused by a single factor which could range from unbalanced humours to miasmas and filth itself. These underlying causes would interact in complex ways with environmental factors and individual predispositions, but, in general terms, different diseases such as plague, cholera, or typhus could all be explained as resulting from a single motive — whatever that might be. That reasoning set the basis for discussions in early chemistry and pharmacology as well. If all diseases ultimately result from the same cause, then it makes sense to search for a single remedy to cure them all: a *panacea* or a *philosopher's stone*. Consequently, conditions that would be categorised differently in the twentieth century could be reasonably seen as near-equivalents two centuries ago.

This is noticeable also in the survival of the therapy and prevention strategies practised from the fourteenth century onwards. Prevention against cholera or typhoid in the nineteenth century involved segregation, quarantine, and flight, practices which were in many instances created and perfected during the plague outbreaks of previous centuries. Although societies around the world and throughout history have intuitively grasped the concept of contagion and have isolated individuals suffering

---

32   Mark Twain, *The Innocents Abroad, or The New Pilgrims Progress* (Hartford: American Publishing Company, 1875), p. 219.

from certain ailments, the first documented evidence of quarantine being enforced as state policy dates from 1377 and belongs to the city of Ragusa (now Dubrovnik), then part of the Venetian Republic.[33] The quarantine policy was a direct result of the challenges posed by the Black Death and the realization that its spread relied heavily on maritime commerce. In subsequent years, Venice would continue to take measures in that direction: the plague hospital (Lazzaretto Vecchio) was adapted in 1423 to house plague victims, a board of health was created in 1485, and health licences (*fedi di sanità*) certifying an individual's provenience from a plague-free zone were implemented in the late sixteenth and early seventeenth centuries.[34] These measures would continue to be used in later periods and are linked to many collective habits adopted during the current pandemic: quarantines, lockdowns, social distancing, or restricted mobility conditioned by negative tests or proof of vaccination. Arguably, current discussions about COVID green passes, individual freedom and state policy have their roots in this period.

Besides that, official recommendations to avoid cholera in the nineteenth century could often be found in previous plague treatises. The report produced by the University of Paris in 1348 suggests people could avoid plague by maintaining simple diets, bypassing stress and anxiety, keeping away from excessive sex and drinking, and purifying the air by burning chamomile, among others. The same advice is propagated time and again during the cholera pandemics, with the sole difference that chamomile should be consumed in tea rather than burned as incense. In this manner, until the last decades of the nineteenth century, there were substantial historical, cultural, and even medical reasons for cholera to be seen as an equivalent of the plague. The perceived likeness kept the memory of the plague alive even in a century in which European outbreaks became rarer and diminished in scale. Regardless of that, for the average person at this place and time, epidemics were, literally, a matter of choice between plague and cholera.

Interestingly, a similar pattern arose in the early months of the coronavirus pandemic when little was known for certain about the virus. There was no agreement at the time on the best therapeutic protocol, and vaccines were still at their earliest stage of development. In these circumstances,

---

33   Gian Franco Gensini, and Magdi H. Yacoub, and Andrea A. Conti, 'The concept of quarantine in history: from plague to SARS', *Journal of Infection*, 49, 2004(4), 257–61 (p. 259).

34   Kristy Wilson Bowers, 'Plague and Developments in Public Health', in Byrne, pp. 424–84.

individuals received the same advice they would have in previous centuries: eat healthfully, stay hydrated, rest and sleep well, avoid stress, and keep away from large groups. Suddenly, the novelty of COVID-19 allowed for the re-emergence of old patterns of interpretation and reaction which were directly linked to cholera and the plague.

If this conclusion seems far-fetched, the Influenza Pandemic offers another case in point. In 1900, Sidney experienced a limited outbreak of bubonic plague — about three hundred confirmed cases — that continued to flare up until 1910. In this decade, Australia reported 1.371 official cases and 535 deaths.[35] Unsurprisingly, the epidemic engendered great concern among the public, so when the new threat of the Spanish Flu emerged in Sidney in late 1918, the population naturally understood the latter in light of the former. Just like cholera a century earlier, newspapers reported sensational accounts conflating the two diseases. In parallel to the Black Death, some families with suffering members marked their houses with flags.[36] The extent of the overlap became manifest when Lucy Taksa collected oral histories in the 1990s. Several interviewees asserted they could recall "the Bubonic Plague" or avowed to have been inoculated against it.[37] One person declared about Influenza: "I always understood it was the same kind of flu that swept Europe, the Black Death in the Middle Ages. I think it was the same kind of thing, it was carried by fleas on rats".[38] Furthermore, the effect was not restricted to Australia since similar accounts were registered by folklorists in the United States during the 1930s. The shoemaker James Hughes professes, for instance:

> D'ya remember the flu thet come the tame a the war? Alwiays a war brengs somethin' an' I alwiays thought thet flu wuzn't jest the flu. It wuz more laike the bumbatic pliague [bubonic plague]. Anywiays a lotta thim thet daied a it

---

35 Bubonic plague, *National Museum of Australia*, 13 March 2020, <https://www.nma.gov.au/defining-moments/resources/bubonic-plague> (last access: March 5th, 2021).

36 Lucy Taksa, 'Plagues, Pandemics and Playback Loops: War-time footing and urgent lessons from history', <https://www.mq.edu.au/__data/assets/pdf_file/0006/972519/Lucy-Taksa-CWF-Critical-Discussion-2020-Plagues-Pandemics-and-Playback-Loops.pdf> (last access: March 5th, 2021).

37 Lucy Taksa, 'The Masked disease: oral history, memory and the Influenza Pandemic, 1918-19', in Kate Darian-Smith and Paula Hamilton, *Memory and history in twentieth century Australia* (Oxford: Oxford University Press, 1994), pp. 79–84.

38 Taksa, 'The Masked disease: oral history, memory and the Influenza Pandemic, 1918-19', in Darian-Smith and Hamilton, p. 88.

tirned black, jest laike thiey wuz said ta heve tirned black in Ireland in '46 an' '47 whin thiey hed the bumbatic pliague thiere. [?][39]

If cholera and influenza could be confused with the plague in the public imagination, why would the coronavirus — which resembles the flu — be treated much differently? The fact that these diseases could be conceived similarly impacted cultural perceptions, habits, and interpretations. One such connection is evident in the current habit of wearing protective masks. When the precaution was called for in the early months of the pandemic, countless articles in the media drew parallels between the new COVID-19 masks and the bird-like masks of plague doctors, indirectly claiming there to be a connection between the two. Although plague masks are easily recognisable today, they are absent from the images representing the plague from the fourteenth to the seventeenth century. In fact, there is very little evidence for their usage. The two earliest treatises to describe and illustrate them are dated 1661 and 1721. The proximity of these dates to the perceived end of the plague outbreaks in Europe underscores that this was a late phenomenon. Moreover, very few masks have survived, and those that did are of dubious provenance. An analysis of two of the masks presented in German museums has shown that they were clumsy, impractical, and, even if possibly authentic, unlikely to have been used during real medical emergencies.[40] When considered together, these elements show how, contrary to common legend, plague masks were not widespread but were used on rare occasions that could very well be ritualistic or commemorative rather than medical — if they were used at all. Thus, there is a genuine possibility that plague masks are, in effect, a cultural construction, a way to imagine the past that started in the seventeenth century and reached the present day.[41]

Yet, even if the current masks are not directly linked to those of plague doctors, they are certainly tied to the plague as a disease. The modern masks emerged during a plague outbreak in Manchuria (northeast China) in 1910.[42] They were created and implemented by Chinese physician and

---

39   Stephanie Hall, 'Stories from the 1918-1919 Influenza Pandemic from Ethnographic Collections', Library of Congress, 15 April 2020, <https://blogs.loc.gov/folklife/2020/04/stories-influenza-pandemic/> (last access: March 5th, 2021).

40   Marion M. Ruisinger, 'Die Pestarztmaske im Deutschen Medizinhistorischen Museum Ingolstadt', *N.T.M.*, 28, (2020), 235–52 (pp. 426–47).

41   Ruisinger, p. 250.

42   Christos Lynteris, 'Plague masks: the visual emergence of anti-epidemic personal protection equipment', *Medical Anthropology*, 37.6 (2018), 442–57.

Cambridge graduate Wu Liande. Contrary to the major practices of the time, Dr. Wu emphasised the airborne spread of pneumonic plague and, as a result, defended the usage of an 'anti-plague mask'. His design was based on that of surgery masks — created just recently, in 1897 — with the addition of further layers for filtration. It was the first time that personal protective equipment was used to control an epidemic and the experiment was soon repeated on a much wider scale during the 1918 Influenza pandemic, before being reimplemented for the present crisis.

4. The Plague metaphors in the times of the Coronavirus

Cholera and influenza were not the only pandemics to invoke images of plague and to conflate them. Comparable ideas surfaced regularly at the start of the AIDS pandemic, just like the Ebola scare of 2014 was used to posit the relevance of studying the plague's history today.[43] In that sense, the recollection of the plague in the times of Coronavirus confirms a historical tendency, even if its causes — as typical of such broad phenomena — are numerous and complex.

Firstly, plague metaphors are powerful and old, even preceding the Black Death itself. They abound in the Bible, where they are often presented along with other scourges. Ezekiel (14:21) speaks of 'sword, famine, wild beasts, and plague' as tantamount, while the damages inflicted by the Four Horsemen of the Apocalypse have been variously interpreted as war, pestilence, and political oppression, among others. In the *First Chronicles* and the *Second Book of Samuel*, David is urged to determine his own damnation: three days of plague, three months of enemy pursuit, or three years of famine. Assuming that the penances are equivalent — God allowing for a choice of personal preference rather than degree of severity — the plague comes across as the worst calamity, accomplishing in days that which famine achieves in years.

For that reason, the plague metaphors are ambivalent enough to be bent in almost any direction. In literature, Pär Lagerkvist's *The Dwarf* (*Dvärgen*, 1944) or Albert Camus' *The Plague* (*La Peste*, 1947) manipulate it to create allegories of Fascism; André Brink utilized it to discuss the apartheid

---

43 Monica H. Green, 'Preface. The Black Death and Ebola: on the value of comparison', in Ead. (ed.), *Pandemic disease in the medieval world: rethinking the black death*, pp. IX–XX.

system in *The Wall of the Plague* (1984); Antonin Artaud invoked it to contextualise his Avant-guard theatre.

Nevertheless, plague metaphors are not the monopoly of artists. As astutely remarked by Susan Sontag, the idea of plague — or cancer for that matter — has the power to unite and to exclude. Since transmissible diseases are invariably seen as coming "from the outside", they create a cultural dichotomy between the *ingroup* and the *outgroup*, between *us* and *them*. Moreover, diseases are considered unnatural incidents which must be dealt with and, if possible, sanitised and eradicated.

It follows that discourses on plague are quite useful politically as a strategy to diffuse attention or unify agendas through fear and common hatred. That was the case in the past and it continues to be the rationale behind much of the populist rhetoric employed during the COVID-19 crisis. In the fourteenth century, the plague was famously blamed on Jews and Lepers. In the sixteenth century, syphilis was first described by physicians as *peste cruelle* ('cruel plague') and *ignota pestis* ('unknown pestilence'); yet, its name was quickly transformed as its identity was reimagined locally in relationship to one's perceived enemies: in France, syphilis was called *le mal de Naples* ('Naples disease'); in Italy, *il mal francese* or the *morbus gallicus* ('the French disease'); in Poland, it was 'the German disease'; in Russia, 'the Polish disease'; in North Africa, 'the Spanish evil'; and, in India, 'the Portuguese evil' or 'the foreigner's disease'.[44] By the same token, cholera was consistently envisaged as *Asiatic cholera* or *Indian cholera* in the nineteenth century, a fact that has even influenced the scientific understanding of the affliction.[45]

Such rhetoric combining epidemics and group identity is, in fact, so common that it can be seen as a cultural habit of its own and one which is amply used at present. The right-wing Brazilian president Jair Bolsonaro, for instance, repeatedly engaged it to create a sense of unity among his supporters when the coronavirus pandemic had just reached Brazil. After consistently attacking science, scientists, and the World Health Organization, Bolsonaro urged his followers to fast to rid Brazil of Coronavirus, a statement which his allies hailed as a saint proclamation.[46] Trump likewise referred to Coronavirus as the "China virus" and "Kung

---

44   Ernest L. Abel, 'Syphilis: The History of an Eponym', *Names, a journal of onomastics*, v. 66, n. 2 (2018), 96–102 (p. 98).

45   Aureo L. Guerios, *Cholera and the Literary Imagination in Europe, 1830-1930*, PhD diss. (Padua: University of Padua, 2021), pp. 41–64.

46   Matheus Teixeira, 'Bolsonaro faz chamado para jejum religioso neste domingo contra coronavírus', Folha de São Paulo, 4 April 2020, <https://www1.folha.uol.

Flu" on numerous occasions in order to channel people's discontent towards a political and economic rival.[47] According to some Italian media, Matteo Salvini, the ex-Minister of the Interior, used information on viral contagion to call for a stop to the arrival of migrants from Africa.[48] In India, Hindu nationalists inculpated Muslims for the crisis.[49]

Once the metaphors of invasive diseases are directed against people, they implicitly point to genocide.[50] Given that illness must be eradicated to relinquish human suffering, by the same token, individuals or groups considered a social plague should disappear in some way or another. Nazism's depiction of Jewish people in *The Eternal Jew* (*Der ewige Jude*, 1940) as syphilitic plague spreaders is an infamous and chilling example of the power of such metaphors and the terrible outcomes they may help achieve. It is no coincidence that, as the elections approached, Donald Trump exacerbated his rhetoric, repeatedly referring to COVID-19 as the plague from China, especially when commenting on the poor economic performance of his late-term.[51] The inflammatory oratory would devolve a little later into wilful attacks on democracy and the endorsement of white supremacist groups.

There are also more mundane reasons for the revisitation and construction of plague memories. One of them is the novelty of the problem. The newness

---

com.br/poder/2020/04/bolsonaro-faz-chamado-para-jejum-religioso-neste-domingo-contra-coronavirus.shtml> (last access: May 27th, 2022).

47   President Trump calls coronavirus kung flu, BBC News, 24 June 2020, <https://www.bbc.com/news/av/world-us-canada-53173436> (last access: March 5th, 2021).

48   Alessandro Massone, 'No, per il nuovo coronavirus non ha alcun senso parlare di allarme-contagio dall'Africa', The Submarine, 5 February 2020, <https://thesubmarine.it/2020/02/05/africa-coronavirus-allarme-contagio-salvini/> (last access: March 5th, 2021).

49   Murali Krishnan, 'Indian Muslims face renewed stigma amid COVID-19 crisis,' Deutsche Welle, 14 May 2020, <https://www.dw.com/en/indian-muslims-face-renewed-stigma-amid-covid-19-crisis/a-53436462> (last access: March 5th, 2021).

50   Susan Sontag, *Illness as Metaphor* (New York: Farrar, Straus and Giroux, 1978), pp. 84–87.

51   Patrick Wintour and Julian Borger, 'Trump attacks China over Covid plague as Xi urges collaboration in virus fight', The Guardian, 22 September 2020, <https://www.theguardian.com/world/2020/sep/22/trump-china-xi-beijing-united-nations> (last access: March 5th, 2021); Eric Loch, '"Before the Plague Came, I Had It Made": Trump Strikes a Doubtful Note in Pennsylvania', The New Yorker, 21 October 2020, <https://www.newyorker.com/news/campaign-chronicles/before-the-plague-came-i-had-it-made-trump-strikes-a-doubtful-note-in-pennsylvania> (last access: March 5th, 2021).

and unfamiliarity of COVID-19 invite old patterns of behaviour and interpretation — as did cholera in the 1830s and influenza in the late 1910s. From a practical point of view, until scientific knowledge is built around the new threat, society is plunged for a period into the pre-modern-medicine era. Even though questions about COVID-19's cause and mechanism of spread were swiftly answered, the lack of therapy and vaccines forced societies all over the world to turn to old plague prevention strategies such as quarantines, social distancing, and masks. These similarities with other pandemic responses in history proportionally diminish as science advances solutions. In the meantime, however, the remembrance of things past arises naturally, and individuals and societies are tempted to re-enact the old habits associated with pre-modern pandemics, among which, the plague prevails.

The same holds for cultural representations. A new threatening disease will only form its own identity and accompanying set of metaphors after familiarity develops. Time is required for that to happen, so, in the meanwhile, old patterns of interpretation prevail. Among these, the plague stands out as the best suited and most spectacular. It would be unfeasible to explain Coronavirus through the lens of other afflictions: cancer metaphors do not address contagiousness appropriately; those of syphilis are too deeply associated with sex and personal retribution; tuberculosis — even if airborne and breath-related — is unsuitably linked to art and refinement. Given that these metaphors ensure disparate interpretations of the health crisis as a whole, they also affect the formation of habits very differently. For example, the belief that tuberculosis was a sort of angelical ailment that targeted those who were too virtuous for earthly existence — women and children above all — allowed for the symptoms of the disease to influence cultural trends such as fashion design and even beauty standards. A case in point is the German philosopher Karl Rosenkranz, who comments in his essay *Aesthetics of Ugliness*:

> But illness is not ugly in cases like phthisis [i.e., tuberculosis], mania, or states of fever, when it gives the organism a transcendent tincture that makes it appear downright ethereal. Emaciation, a burning gaze, the pale or fever-blushed cheeks of the patient can even make the essence of the spirit more directly visible. [...] Who has not seen on a deathbed a virgin or youth who, as a victim of consumption, offered a truly transfigured sight! [...] A convalescent is a sight for the gods![52]

---

52   Karl Rosenkranz, *Aesthetics of Ugliness: a critical edition*, trans. by Andrei Pop and Mechtild Widrich (London: Bloomsbury Publishing, 2015), pp. 45–46.

As shown by Carolyn Day, the positive metaphors associated with tuberculosis amazingly turned its outward manifestations (pale skin, thin bodies, red lips, etc.) into desirable traits.[53] This led, in turn, to changes in habits of dress and behaviour. Victorian makeup, for instance, welcomed the emaciated appearance of consumptive patients by trying to mimic their perceived pale faces and red lips and cheeks — an appeal which can also be found in many paintings by the Pre-Raphaelites.

This shows how the metaphors of tuberculosis are built very differently from those of the plague and, therefore, influence habits and cultural interpretations in equally disparate ways. The plague metaphors are best suited for scenarios in which a disease is new and unfamiliar, spreads quickly through the population, acts swiftly, is mortal to some degree and does not become chronicle or debilitating for life — all characteristics which also apply to COVID-19. Beyond the plague, few illnesses share all these characteristics. As we have seen, cholera and influenza behaved thus at some point in history, but they were themselves understood at the time through the plague's lenses rather than engendering a set of metaphors of their own. Perhaps, the sole event which could rival the plague as a viable metaphor is the great dying of the native peoples of the Americas in the sixteenth century. As previously mentioned, the deadly combination of diseases brought along with the conquistadores is akin to the Black Death at many levels: an enormous death toll, high contagiousness, rapid proliferation, and societal collapse. These features notwithstanding, the dismal effects of the Colombian exchange are not sufficiently known by the general population to give birth to prompt comparisons. In addition, its historical unravelling is very complex, involving a great number of afflictions and other synchronous phenomena (violent expansion, enslavement, evangelism, cultural imperialism), all of which are equally intricate in their own right and which, once again, diffuse the already scarce public attention. The great dying of the sixteenth century certainly led to collapse, but one which is imagined within Sontag's dichotomy of *ingroup* versus *outgroup* as something that afflicted only *them* and sparred *us*. This perceived immunity precludes the metaphor to be viable for *us* — whoever that might be.

Beyond that, there is one characteristic that, in my opinion, is fundamental to our contemporary intake on the plague as a way of understanding the present challenge: the simplicity of the plague narrative.

---

53   Carolyn Day, *Consumptive chic: a history of beauty, fashion, and disease* (London: Bloomsbury Publishing, 2017).

On collective memory, the Black Death surfaces inexplicably as a force of nature, threatening humans with annihilation for no reason whatsoever or, alternatively, due to collective sin. It reigned terror for four centuries, only to allegedly disappear in the eighteenth century — as mysteriously as it first broke out. This simple story offers two convenient advantages. Firstly, it invokes old interpretation patterns of disasters as heavenly punishment, something that allows *us* to blame *them* for the tragedy, and, concomitantly, to look at *ourselves* as victims – for what could we do against such a massive event? Especially if sent by God? If we did not look back to the plague metaphors, we would perhaps be forced to gaze into the real reasons behind the Coronavirus pandemic: climate change, imminent ecological collapse, staggering environmental pollution, overpopulation, unsustainable industrial growth, wealth inequality, and so forth. Each one of these issues is formidable and convoluted on its own terms. There is no easy and simple solution to any of them, nor will there ever be. However, since complexity often fails our need to explain phenomena in simple terms imbued with intents and purposes, it is uncomfortable to live with such a wide range of causes. Many would find the idea that there is no ultimate meaning behind the Coronavirus pandemic — apart from being a sign of a world out of balance — assuredly daunting. There *must be* meaning behind an event that is at the root of so much suffering; if there is not, then it is necessary to invent one. The old plague metaphors fulfil this cultural and psychological need through a coherent and simple narrative. Interestingly, much of the meaning attributed to the plague is pre-scientific and is constructed to cope with a tragedy that is enormously superior to our own. The dissonances are cast aside, however, overwritten by the demand for a simple, unified narrative.

On top of that, the plague experience offers an opportunity to contemplate annihilation from a different perspective. Since 1945, the idea of a human-induced apocalypse has been looming in the public mind. Between the 1950s and 1980s, it took the form of nuclear war, and, as that threat subsided, it gave way to the menace of global warming and climate change. The more recent anxieties are also accompanied by predictions of the emergence of zoonotic diseases and pathogens resistant to antibiotics. In this context, looking back to the plague experience allows us to take a paradoxical stance. From one side, it helps us acknowledge and understand the real possibility that humans might cease to exist in the future — or at least that civilisation as we know it might have to be reinvented completely. Yet, on the opposite side, it also allows us to find relief and to enjoy a happy ending of sorts. Since the plague narrative is shaped in terms of the disappearance of a once-mighty menace, it presents us with a paramount example of human endurance and everlasting triumph.

Nearly all cultural and artistic representations of a post-apocalyptic world point to some type of renewal — or at least the hope of it. This is manifest at the end of Camus' *The Plague*: although we know not for how long the truce will last, at least for a time the world is saved. Celebratory conclusions such as this one are found in countless films and novels ranging from Defoe's *A Journal of the Plague Year* (1722) to the Hollywood blockbuster *Contagion* (2011). Even when nearly all of humanity has been exterminated, many post-apocalyptic texts reach the end with a flint of hope and renewal. This is the case in Mary Shelley's *The Last Man* (1826), whose protagonist roams the planet in search of another Eve to re-establish humanity; or in *The Near End of the World* (*O Quase Fim do Mundo*, 2008) by the contemporary Angolan writer Pepetela, in which a small group of survivors decide to repopulate the world out of Africa for the second time.

When used in relation to the Coronavirus, the plague metaphors permit us to collectively see what we already believe: collective human tenacity in the face of adversity will eventually — and perhaps almost inevitably — triumph over the challenges, despite their monumentality. In the end, humans always prevail, and if the world is left in ruins, the survivors will somehow rebuild civilisation anew. Hence, the plague metaphors can paradoxically offer emotional relief, offering on occasion a form of Aristotelian purification (*katharsis*). At least as far as narratives go.

DAVID VINCENT

THE EPIDEMIC AND THE PANDEMIC
Loneliness and Covid-19

1. Before the pandemic there was an epidemic

Loneliness as a negative form of solitude emerged as a concept two hundred years ago.[1] By the second half of the twentieth century it was becoming a public responsibility. The creation of the welfare state in 1948, committed successive governments not only to maintaining the health of the population but also to caring for the increasing numbers of elderly citizens. The longer people lived, the more likely it was that they would encounter long periods of widowhood, the more they moved into their own homes, the greater the danger that they would lose the support of their children, whose numbers were also falling. It was far from clear that the public finances could afford the bill, and studies began to appear attempting to calculate the scale of the challenge.[2]

More recently there has been an added concern that the post-industrial economy was dissolving what was left of traditional communities, threatening a wholesale erosion of inter-personal relations. It was feared that more and more people were unable to make meaningful connections with each other. The historian Keith Snell conducted a large-scale literature review in 2016 and concluded that 'Loneliness is now widely diagnosed as a modern "epidemic" or "plague"'[3] Following a report published by the Jo Cox Commission on Loneliness (named in honour of a recently murdered

---

1   Fay Bound Alberti, 'This "Modern Epidemic": Loneliness as an Emotion Cluster and a Neglected Subject in the History of Emotions', *Emotion Review*, 10, 3 (2018), 242–54 (p. 1); Fay Bound Alberti, *A Biography of Loneliness* (Oxford: Oxford University Press, 2019), pp. 17–39.
2   Jeremy Tunstall, *Old and Alone. A Sociological Study of Old People* (London: Routledge and Kegan Paul, 1966), pp. 1–2.
3   K. D. M. Snell, 'Agendas for the Historical Study of Loneliness and Lone Living', *The Open Psychology Journal*, 8 (Supplement 2-M2), (2015), 61–70 (p. 62).

Member of Parliament),[4] the Conservative Government of Theresa May launched an official strategy to combat loneliness in England in October 2018, entitled *A Connected Society*, and appointed the world's first 'loneliness minister.'[5] There have since been changes in the postholder, and the responsibility is now exercised by a junior minister in the House of Lords.[6] Two official reviews of the strategy have been conducted, and Scotland and Wales have published their own action programmes. Boris Johnson's administration has not allowed itself to be distracted by Covid-19. The most recent review, published in January 2021 at the height of the third wave of infection, committed it to reducing stigma and ensuring that loneliness is embedded in policy making.[7]

The persisting attachment of the term 'epidemic' to loneliness indicated the scale of the moral panic. At one level it was a just a metaphor. It inferred that loneliness was a large and negative event. If, for instance, we say that someone received an 'avalanche of complaints,' we do not mean literally that they were covered in a pile of rocks and ice, just that they experienced a great deal of criticism.

The second implication was more specific. It reflected an attempt to medicalise a social condition. This discourse was a function of the way that political change works in a democracy. Pressure groups and concerned scientists have since the 1950s gradually compelled governments to intervene in a growing range of private behaviours which have demonstrable medical consequences. The campaigners against loneliness appropriated the narrative of a public health emergency, claiming that the condition was the equivalent smoking fifteen cigarettes a day or having too large a waistline. What Judith Shulevitz has termed "the lethality of loneliness" became the subject of widespread public commentary.[8] The list of possible outcomes grew rapidly. By the time the British government launched its loneliness

---

4   The Jo Cox Commission on Loneliness, *Combatting loneliness one conversation at a time: A call to action* (London: 2017).
5   HM Government, *A connected society. A strategy for tackling loneliness – laying the foundations for change* (London: Department for Digital, Culture, Media and Sport, October, 2018). On the background to the document see, David Vincent, *A History of Solitude* (Cambridge: Polity, 2020), pp. 220–21.
6   Baroness Diana Barran.
7   For a survey of government policies on loneliness since 2017 see, Philip Loft, *Tackling Loneliness* (House of Commons Briefing Paper, 22 February 2021).
8   Judith Shulevitz, 'The Lethality of Loneliness', The New Republic, 27 May 2013, 21–29.

strategy, the condition was associated with almost every contemporary medical crisis. 'Its health impact' claimed *The Connected Society*,

> is thought to be on a par with other public health priorities like obesity or smoking. Research shows that loneliness is associated with a greater risk of inactivity, smoking and risk-taking behaviour; increased risk of coronary heart disease and stroke; an increased risk of depression, low self-esteem, reported sleep problems and increased stress response; and with cognitive decline and an increased risk of Alzheimer's.[9]

The influential American psychologists John Cacioppo and Stephanie Cacioppo claimed in an article in *The Lancet* in 2018 that loneliness was a 'contagious' condition affecting one third of the of the population of industrial countries.[10] The discourse has thrown renewed attention on the search for a loneliness pill.[11] Stephanie Cacioppo is continuing work on isolating a pharmacological treatment for social isolation.[12] Another research group is investigating the prescription of oxytocin for loneliness sufferers. Whether these pills are a self-sufficient remedy or part of a psychotherapy treatment, the prospects for the pharmaceutical companies are immense.

Critics of this diagnosis focused on both the numbers and the causal relationship. Christina Victor and colleagues concluded in 2003 that 'there appears to be little strong or compelling evidence to suggest that we are either experiencing an epidemic of loneliness in old age or that rates of loneliness have increased markedly over time.'[13] Although there is no consistent measure of acute loneliness since the second world war, studies of the elderly suggest that the baseline figure is around five per cent. A recent review of the evidence concludes that there is 'no empirical support for the fact that loneliness is increasing, let alone spreading at

---

9   HM Government, p. 18.
10   John T. Cacioppo and Stephanie Cacioppo, 'The growing problem of loneliness', *The Lancet*, 391 (10119) (3 February 2018), 426. This approach is discussed in greater length in John T. Cacioppo and William Patrick, *Loneliness. Human Nature and the Need for Social Connection* (New York: W.W. Norton, 2008), p. 5.
11   <https://www.theguardian.com/lifeandstyle/2020/aug/06/loneliness-cure-pill-research-scientists?CMP=share_btn_link> (last access: November 13th, 2021).
12   Her collaborator and husband John Cacioppo died in 2018.
13   Christina Victor, Ann Bowling, John Bond and Sasha Scambler, 'Loneliness, Social Isolation, and Living Alone in Later Life,' *Research Findings* no 17, Growing Older Programme. Economic and Social Research Council (April 2003), 1–4. See also, G. Clare Wenger and others, 'Social Isolation and Loneliness in Old Age: Review and Model Refinement', *Ageing and Society*, 16 (1996), 333–58 (p. 336).

epidemic rates.'[14] Whilst there were a range of physical and psychological conditions which might contribute to loneliness, the condition could not be caught by exposure to other sufferers. Conversely the health consequences of loneliness were too diffuse and too related to broader experiences of depression to constitute an identifiable pathology.

With the arrival of a real medical epidemic, re-labelled a pandemic as soon as its global reach became apparent, it seemed unlikely that this frame of reference could persist. Covid-19 made all too apparent what a lethal infectious disease really looked like. Nevertheless, the term continued to be applied to loneliness in public conversation. At the height of the third wave of Covid-19 in Britain, government initiatives in the field were still being discussed as if a separate loneliness epidemic was continuing alongside the pandemic. It was reported in December 2020, that: "A volunteer phone call service for older and vulnerable social housing residents and a homemade Christmas food delivery service are among a number of initiatives being singled out for praise as the government announces a £7.5m fund to tackle the epidemic of loneliness in England."[15] In Parliament, the leader of the Social Democrats, Ed Davey, suggested that the lockdown had 'created a silent epidemic of loneliness.'[16] On the day this paragraph was written, the All Party Parliamentary Group on Loneliness issued a report demanding action to tackle a 'loneliness emergency' that the pandemic has exacerbated by denying people contact with family and friends.[17]

There were strong *prima facie* grounds for assuming that Covid-19 and actions taken by the Government to combat it would worsen the pre-existing incidence of loneliness. The Ministerial Forward to the second review of the Loneliness Strategy painted a grim picture:

---

14   Esteban Ortiz-Ospina, 'Is there a loneliness epidemic?' (University of Oxford / Our World in Data, December 11, 2019), np.

15   <https://www.theguardian.com/global/commentisfree/2020/dec/20/pandemic-behavior-coronavirus-plague-defoe?CMP=Share_iOSApp_Other> (last access: November 13th, 2021).

16   <https://www.theguardian.com/society/2020/dec/05/poll-reveals-scale-of-home-alone-christmas-in-the-uk-this-year?> (last access: November 13th, 2021). See also Emma Beddington, 'There is an epidemic of loneliness', <https://www.theguardian.com/commentisfree/2021/mar/22/we-are-all-either-desperately-lonely-or-desperate-for-alone-time-which-are-you.> (last access: November 13th, 2021).

17   <https://www.theguardian.com/society/2021/mar/24/post-covid-loneliness-emergency-mps> (last access: November 13th, 2021).

The measures to control the virus have had a devastating effect on our collective mental health and wellbeing. Their particular cruelty has been to deprive us of the very thing that makes us human and gives meaning to our lives — our physical connection with other people. We have missed the everyday social interactions that add color to our days, whether it's sharing food around a table, or meeting friends.[18]

The thirty-one percent of the UK population who were living alone in the second decade of the twenty-first century would be deprived of many of the devices that made their isolation bearable.[19] For long periods it was no longer possible to go shopping other than for basic necessities. They were trapped in their flats or houses, unable to eat out, meet in coffee shops or take holidays. Visits to relations and friends were more or less impossible depending on the state of the lockdown regulations and wholly forbidden for those with pre-existing health conditions.

2. Isolation and desolation?

The growing army of the bereaved threatened further isolation. In the debate over the scale and effect of loneliness it has long been recognised that what Peter Townsend described as the 'desolation' caused by the loss of an intimate partner in old age held the greatest danger to physical and emotional wellbeing.[20] Grief professionals have conventionally worked on the basis of at least five seriously bereaved people for every death.[21] Recent research on the pandemic in the United States suggests that the multiplier is nearer to nine.[22] On that basis, the current COVID-19 mortality rate in Britain of 126,000 would generate over a million suffering relatives and

---

18 Department for Digital, Culture, Media & Sport, *Loneliness Annual Report: the second year* (22 January 2021), Forward.

19 K. D. M. Snell, 'The rise of living alone and loneliness in history', *Journal of Social History*, 42, 1 (2017), 2–28 (p. 9); Ray Hall, Philip E. Ogden and Catherine Hill, 'The Pattern and Structure of One-Person Households in England and Wales and France', *International Journal of Population Geography*, 3 (1997), 161–81 (pp. 162–63).

20 Peter Townsend, *The Family Life of Old People* (London: Routledge and Kegan Paul, 1957), p. 182.

21 Julia Samuel, *Grief Works. Stories of Life, Death and Surviving* (London: Penguin Life, 2017), p. xii.

22 Ashton M. Verdery and others, 'Tracking the reach of COVID-19 kin loss with a bereavement multiplier applied to the United States', *Proceedings of the National Academy of Sciences of the United States*, 117, 30 (July 28, 2020), 17695–17701.

close friends. The circumstances surrounding the death of a loved one were likely to deepen and prolong the grief of those left behind. The sudden onset of the lethal phase of COVID-19, the isolation controls imposed in intensive care units, and the severe restrictions imposed on funerals and wakes made it almost impossible to conduct the long-established rituals that accompanied dying and death. Those left behind were in a state of shock, unable to come to terms with their loss or find solace in the company of others.

The pre-Covid-19 crisis over loneliness, and the predicted intensification of the condition once it commenced, meant that from the outset systematic efforts were made to measure its incidence. In March 2020, The Office for National Statistics (ONS), the leading Government agency for quantifying both the incidence and the consequences of the pandemic, converted its monthly Opinions and Lifestyle Survey into a weekly report. It asked a balanced national sample of 6,000 adults the basic question, "How Often do you feel Lonely?"[23] At the same time a research programme was devised, funded and launched with remarkable speed by a team led by Daisy Fancourt at University College London. The UCL Nuffield COVID-19 Study (UCL) recruited a panel of 70,000 people to respond to inquiries about their mental health and wellbeing. On the issue of loneliness, it employed a shortened version of the Revised UCLA Loneliness Scale, the most widely used American measure of the condition. Both sets of statistical analysis were operational from the moment the first lockdown began on March 23th, 2020, and have continued in an unbroken sequence to the current day. As was the case with the Mass Observation studies in the Second World War, a national crisis has led to a major increase in public knowledge about Britain's state of mind.

Despite the differences in sampling and categorisation, the two contemporary surveys have generated almost identical pictures of variations in loneliness during the pandemic. Whilst the incidence of infection, hospitalisation and deaths have displayed a roller-coaster of rises and falls over twelve months, the graph of loneliness is almost flat. The UCL measure stood at just under five in March 2020 and is still at that level. It fell slightly during the relaxation of controls in September 2020 and rose a little with the third lockdown in January 2021 before returning to the initial figure. Similarly, the ONS figure for 'often / always lonely', the category where potential mental or physical harm takes place, described

---

23   The response rate was around 72%.

a largely horizontal line across the period. It stood at 6% when the first lockdown was imposed in the last week of March 2020, falling back to 5% during the summer, rising to 7% in the second lockdown in the late autumn, and to 8% in the third lockdown in January 2021, and back to 7% as the hospitalisation and death rates began to be driven down by vaccinations in March 2021.[24] A percentage point represents just over half a million adults in the UK and the changes are not to be disregarded altogether. Nonetheless they remain a pale reflection of the medical and regulatory dramas taking place over the same period.

The most illuminating feature of the statistical tables is the range of variables. On the whole the older and more prosperous and those living in rural areas were a little less at risk of loneliness. The major difference was in self-reported disabilities. The healthy had an 'often/always' loneliness level of only 2.8% in the 8-18 July, 2020, ONS sample, compared with an overall figure of 6.2%. By contrast the disabled displayed a level five times higher at 14.5%. Separate categories of impairment had still higher scores — 19.7% for vision, 15.8% for mobility, 21.7% for learning, 24.7% for mental health. It is not difficult to comprehend why these conditions should discourage or prevent levels of social interaction which individuals wish to undertake, or why they should make the experience of being alone so much more painful. There may also be a reverse causal flow, with, for instance, mental health problems exacerbated by a lack of human contact. The returns suggest that in many cases loneliness is a second order feature of systemic failings in health and social care facilities.[25]

Across the population as a whole, however, what has to be explained is not the scale of change in the incidence of loneliness during the pandemic, but its relative absence. There are several factors involved. In the first place the performance of the loneliness graphs is very similar to that of other emotions tracked by the ONS and UCL surveys. Happiness, life satisfaction, anxiety and depression all follow much the same trajectory over the period. The only graph that even began to match the scale of change in the infection and mortality figures is that of anxiety over food supplies,

---

24   For a full summary of ONS data on loneliness during the pandemic, see <https://www.ons.gov.uk/peoplepopulationandcommunity/wellbeing/articles/mappinglonelinessduringthecoronaviruspandemic/2021-04-07.> (last access: November 13th, 2021).

25   <https://www.ons.gov.uk/peoplepopulationandcommunity/healthandsocialcare/disability/datasets/coronavirusandthesocialimpactsondisabledpeopleingreatbritainmay2020> (last access: November 13th, 2021).

which fell steeply from 60% to around 5% during the first few months, but then has shown no further change as the supermarkets introduce efficient online deliveries.[26] The pattern of response raises questions of national character which can only be answered by a broader international survey. It is tempting to suppose that what we are seeing is a manifestation of the phlegmatic character of British society, resistant to almost any scale of national excitement.

3. *The role of devices and community organisations*

More specifically, the figures were a consequence not so much of a stasis as a capacity to adapt to new circumstances. Much of the commentary on the social consequences of the pandemic assumes a population entering the lockdown bereft of the skills required to endure the new circumstances. In reality, the Covid-19 community inherited material assets and structures of behaviour for coping with social isolation that were adapted to meet the imposed restrictions. The population living alone, mostly by choice, has increased substantially since the Second World War, in Britain and in other western countries. There has not been a commensurate growth in acute loneliness because devices have been found to enable people to enjoy rather than endure their own company.[27] Contact with friends and relatives has been maintained through the technology of mass communication — correspondence, the telephone which became the most popular mode of connecting with others in the 1970s, and finally the internet which added another layer to the ecosystem of interpersonal connections. The television and later digital devices increased the range of domestic entertainments. Homes became more spacious and better lit and heated, permitting a wider range of hobbies and pastimes. Older forms of single-player amusements, such as crosswords or solitaire were supplemented by a range of online games. Then there was gardening. On this over-crowded island, long after the invention of high-rise living, seven out of eight households still occupy in a property with a fragment of nature attached to it. For the elderly the proportion of those with access to private outdoor space is even higher at 92%.[28]

---

26   UCL data.
27   Vincent, pp. 153–81.
28   <https://www.ons.gov.uk/economy/environmentalaccounts/articles/oneineightbritishhouseholdshasnogarden/2020-05-14.> (last access: November 13th, 2021).

The delayed but abrupt imposition of a lockdown in England on March 24, 2020, caused a rebalancing of activities. Some forms of voluntary activity, for instance, were prohibited by the regulations, others grew in response to new sets of needs, making use of digital media and permitted transport. A Mass Observation diarist, found that his round of endeavours both contracted and expanded:

> I am active voluntarily in the Parish Council, local history and museum society, Women's Institute, Church choir and Peterborough Cathedral — though the last three of these aren't happening at the moment —. I have zero hour contracts as a tour guide for Vivacity, the cultural trust for Peterborough, and also as an Operations Assistant helping with events at Peterborough Cathedral. This year I started volunteering at Peterborough Food Bank, run by the Trussell Trust and Kingsgate Church.[29]

Many of the community organisations that both supported the lonely and provided a means of connecting them with other people ceased to operate during the pandemic. Regular meetings in parish halls and other venues were no longer possible. In their place were structures of assistance of varying degrees of formality that gave a sense of purpose to the fit and active who were otherwise trapped in their homes, and at the same time provided crucial assistance to those especially vulnerable to infection. The baseline of these practices was the instinctive support by younger family members of older relatives living nearby in the neighbourhood. Thus, for instance a Welsh couple added to their supermarket bill:

> We went shopping for my wife's aunt. Into Tesco Neath Abbey then up to Bryncoch. She left the gate to the garden open so we were able to drop her shopping on the doorstep and sit at the garden table where she brought us a cuppa — keeping the 2 metres distancing... nice to have a chat and good for her I would think as she lives alone.[30]

The voluntary provision of the necessities of life for those who had fallen through the widening gaps in the welfare state had been growing in scale during the decade before the pandemic. Now it was adapted to the new circumstances, making use of the internet to form ad hoc foodbanks. A housewife in her forties donated her time and energy to assist those finding difficulty gaining access to the necessities of life:

29   Mass Observation, 12 May 2020. MT_2020_292.
30   Mass Observation, *Covid Diaries from Non Mass Observers*. 24 April CV19_45.

I have been one of the volunteers from our road since lockdown began, the need being much greater now that people can't visit to collect food themselves. The woman on our road who organised and set up our street WhatsApp group, volunteers there every week and had begun working there more regularly since she couldn't do her 'normal' job during lockdown. There are about 4 or 5 of us (with cars) in our road's group who do deliveries throughout Southwark during the week and I spent just over 2 hours doing deliveries to 5 different households today.[31]

There was a range of means whereby the able-bodied pooled their endeavours to assist those finding it difficult to gain access to the necessities of life. At the same time there was a crucial difference across the population between the locked down and the locked in. Gardeners found a renewed pleasure in plants, and in birdsong made more audible by the temporary cessation in road noise. Then there was the world beyond the garden gate. The short answer to the question of what the British people did during the pandemic is that they went for walks. For centuries, largely unnoticed by historians of leisure, the basic recreation of the mass of the population was stepping out of doors and strolling in nearby lanes, fields or, from the later nineteenth century onwards, municipal parks.[32] At weekends, with the advent of mass transport, there might be excursions to more distant countryside. It was the basic means of escaping the press of company in overcrowded homes, either to enjoy your own company or meet with friends and lovers. The innovation of the lockdown was that this most informal of activities was now legally recognised. It was the one exception to the requirement to stay indoors except for essential shopping, medical assistance and key-working. And in the early weeks of the crisis, the sun shone. A sixty-five-year-old, living alone, found vast pleasure in the world outside:

It's a fabulous spring. I've fallen in love with trees this year, I hadn't realised what a fantastic array of flowers they have; many are small, green and insignificant, but lots are very fragrant. I suppose you just need time to appreciate these things, which, thanks to lockdown is something I currently have. I've walked every day during lockdown, whatever the weather, mostly by the canal and river, in the Riverside Park, the playing fields, round by the crematorium grounds and the old paper mill.[33]

---

31   Mass Observation, 12 May 2020. MT_2020_398.
32   The best survey of this practice remains. Morris Marples, *Shanks's Pony. A Study of Walking* (London: J. M. Dent, 1959). See also Vincent, *Solitude*, pp. 31–70.
33   Mass Observation, 12 May 2020. MT_2020_417.

Those who had dogs were compelled to follow a daily routine, and there was a marked increase in the purchase and thus the price of canine pets, both for the company they provided and the exercise they facilitated.

The more energetic jogged or rode bicycles, and at home there was an increased enthusiasm for bodily fitness regimes, facilitated by a rapid growth in video courses, most notably the daily workouts led by Joe Wicks. Participation was not confined to those seeking to enhance already toned bodies. By these means a woman who was widowed shortly before the pandemic sought to maintain a balance between her continuing bereavement and a life of purposeful solitude. She explained

> Life in lockdown is a solitary experience. It is lonely but curiously I've managed to stay fairly cheerful. It helps that I've had 18 months to adjust to living alone (my husband died unexpectedly in August 2018) and enjoy my own company… Routine is helpful and exercise essential. Having a dog means I always walk every day and have now added in a daily Pilates session.[34]

As with many others, she also used the internet to keep her mind fit: "I used to do a class twice a week before lockdown and was fortunate to have a tutor who has set up Skype sessions so that we can continue at home. This is really motivating."[35]

The range of means by which those living alone sought to resist their isolation is exemplified by an eighty-five-year-old widow in Brighton, who contributed a long diary to Mass Observation. She was recovering from a stroke and not entirely steady of her feet, but she was determined to make the most of her circumstances. She kept as fit as she could by taking regular walks and following a twelve-minute work-out with Mr Motivator on You Tube. As with almost everyone confined to their homes, she was critically dependent on the telephone and the internet for connections with both her neighbourhood, her further-flung family, and wider sources of information, support and entertainment:

> Two WhatsApp groups have been started, one for fun and the other useful, shopping for each other etc. The family also has such a group — my three sons and their partners and my step-daughter and her husband, and a grandson. The phone rings constantly, often with offers of help.[36]

---

34 Mass Observation, 12 May, 2020. MT_2020_124.
35 Mass Observation, 12 May, 2020. MT_2020_124.
36 Mass Observation, *Covid Diaries from Non Mass Observers*. 14 April 2020. CV19_17.

She had already retired before the world began to communicate through screens and keyboards, and from time to time needed the help of one of her sons to help her with the technology. "The young", she noted, "do find it hard sometimes to understand how difficult we find the digital stuff."[37] But she persisted, and former face-to-face activities were adapted to meet her needs. Her mind was still alert, and a mathematics course she had been following in weekly University of the Third Age classes was transferred to Zoom. Before the lockdown, one of her most valued if perverse activities was involvement in the local Methodist church:

> In normal times I have quite a lot to do with them, despite my being an atheist. They do a lot of good work and are very friendly and community minded. They are amused at my description of myself as being an atheist Methodist. I miss their company. The teddy bears are to put in boxes to children in the third world.[38]

However she kept making teddy bears after she had put aside her daily crossword, and in turn the church found ways of maintaining its community. The diary notes:

> Emerged from the shower having washed my hair when the phone rang. Long conversation with a very pleasant woman who helps with the Wednesday old people's lunch I normally go to at the Methodist church… She is ringing everyone who attends in turn to make sure they are ok. It's so warming to know there are so many people who care about one's welfare.[39]

As with most people recording their experiences, there was little that was entirely novel about her lockdown life. Rather, with the help of others, she adapted old practices to meet new circumstances. In doing so she neither escaped nor was overwhelmed by her circumstances as a bereaved elderly woman. 'I think most widows are lonely much of the time,' she observed, 'but I am no more lonely than usual, though I miss my many regular activities.'[40] It was not that she moved up and down a quantitative

---

37   Mass Observation, *Covid Diaries from Non Mass Observers*. 2 May, 2020. CV19_17.

38   Mass Observation, *Covid Diaries from Non Mass Observers*. 14 April, 2020. CV19_17.

39   Mass Observation, *Covid Diaries from Non Mass Observers*. 7 May, 2020. CV19_17.

40   Mass Observation, *Covid Diaries from Non Mass Observers*. 14 April, 2020. CV19_17.

scale of less to more loneliness, but rather that in host of complex ways the relation between her sociable and her isolated life changed its form.

Whilst for the population at large there were increases in efforts to avoid being alone, so also, and sometimes for the same people, there were alterations in the desire to withdraw from company. Solitude in its positive form, what its first modern theorist described as "a tendency to self-collection and freedom,"[41] became increasingly desirable in accommodation crowded with home-working adults and home-schooling children. The condition in the modern era is not seen as a threat to public health and therefore has never been counted. However, during the pandemic, the UCL project twice asked its panel to list the activities that were most missed. In May 2020, almost a third reported a longing to have time on their own and in February 2001 over a fifth.

A leading characteristic of a pandemic is that history is expressed in numbers. Every day reliable national and international bodies issue figures of infections and deaths. This does not mean that the impact on interpersonal relations can be adequately expressed in the same way. It is rather that patterns of human interactions were changed as new pressures were negotiated and new solutions found. Whilst there were victims of intense loneliness, for many more the experience of being alone was just a variation in the journey through life, making the most of both time alone and time in company.

---

41   Johann Zimmerman, *Solitude Considered with Respect to its Dangerous Influence Upon the Mind and Heart* (London: C. Dilly, 1798), p. 21.

CARLA PETROCELLI

TECHNOLOGY IN THE TIME OF PANDEMICS
Digitalization in Crisis Contexts

During one of his usual daily briefings on the COVID-19 emergency in April 2020, New Jersey governor Phil Murphy surprised his viewers with an unusual request: he was looking for coders who knew COBOL, a now obsolete programming language used in unemployment application management systems.

The systems were unable to support the sudden influx of unemployment requests spurred by business closures, staff cuts, and distancing measures. Between the end of March and the first week of April, for example, more than 362,000 New Jersey residents applied for unemployment, generating an overload of the old IBM mainframes on which this software was installed back in the 1980s. Of course, with the tens of thousands of COVID-19 cases at the time, this concern about the obsolescence of computer systems seemed ridiculous, but Governor Murphy was still forced to make this request publicly, given the criticality of the situation.

COBOL (COmmon Business Oriented Language) is now more than six decades old. Surviving all eras and trends – including the Cold War and the rise of the Internet – it is a programming language that remains incredibly popular: in the United States it is used in public administration but also for the management of some federal government agencies, such as the Department of Veterans Affairs, the Department of Justice, and the Social Security Administration. Proposed by mathematic Grace Murray Hopper, it was the first standardized programming language not tied to specific hardware and dedicated to solving economic and financial problems. Her concept of *open source* or "free engineering" can be considered a kind of prophetic anticipation of one of the most interesting innovations introduced in the field of scientific research. As early as 1952, Hopper had referred to the tools and techniques of compilation to allow a simpler method of writing program lines translated automatically into binary language. Her strong belief that the exchange of information strengthened knowledge led her to experiment with a method that later became fundamental to modern information technology: distributed information.[1]

In times of crisis in the US and elsewhere, remedial measures have had to be taken to update these old systems. Just think of the emergency of the year 2000, or the so-called *millennium bug*, caused by the uncertainty that the date of the new millennium would cause cascading errors in all the computer systems of the world. Legions of programmers were specifically hired to correct the code and to avoid the speculated possibility of total economic collapse.

The unprecedented surge in unemployment applications in 2020 thus created a demand for programmers still capable of modifying the old software the application system runs on. Most universities no longer offer courses in COBOL programming, opting to teach about it in computer history courses instead. "There was a period of 20 years where people were sure COBOL was dead, so there was nobody teaching it, nobody learning it," says J. Ray Scott, a professor at Carnegie Mellon University and one of the few who still teaches COBOL today.[2]

To deal with this emergency, the giant IBM took action to find or train other programmers with an initiative aimed at teaching COBOL. This "nostalgia operation" was far from simple; it was realized that the new levers to be put in place should have been in sustained number. According to an estimate made by IBM, there were in fact about 220 billion COBOL code lines still in use in the banking and financial sectors, but also and above all in public administration. In order to evangelize millennials, IBM decided to offer a complete course on the programming language, totally free, hoping to quickly raise a new generation of COBOL coders. In addition, the company also set up a forum open to both old and new programmers, a space in which veteran coders, retired programmers, and students could exchange ideas and solutions to deal with the problem.

Did it take a pandemic for public administration to finally start updating its hardware and software to ensure it performed efficiently for citizens?

---

1   See Henry Tropp, 'Grace Hopper. The youthful teacher of us all', *Abacus*, 2, 1984, 7—18; Carla Petrocelli, *Il computer è donna. Eroine geniali e visionarie che hanno fatto la storia dell'informatica* (Bari: Edizioni Dedalo, 2019), pp. 31–52.

2   Scott today works at the Pittsburg Supercomputer Center as Director of Systems and Operations. Patrick Thibodeau, Member of the Commission. Should Universities Offer Cobol Classes?, Computerworld, 8 April 2013, <https://www.computerworld.com/article/2496360/should-universities-offer-cobol-classes-.html> (last access: November 15th, 2021).

And was this pandemic necessary for us to discover the importance of a connected society?

1. *Flockless men*

As human beings we need the group; without a flock we die. If deprived of contact, we physically and mentally perish. Yet, in the case of this serious epidemic, common living has created a conflict with the need to stem the spread of the virus. In accepting exceptional measures, we have also taken on an aesthetic of distancing and urbanization typical of eastern countries: face masks, bicycles, scooters, and relationships without direct contact have undoubtedly changed the way we look at the world, leading to an inevitable surge in the use of digital technologies.

Between Skype, Zoom, WhatsApp, Virtual Private Networks (VPN), smart-working, distance learning, e-commerce, and social networks, the months we spent in front of a screen made us quickly realize the potential, but also the limits, of this type of communication. The 'digital life' seemed just as consistent and real as traditional life, almost as if there was some continuity between our online and offline identities. It is as if there had been a kind of 'invasion of the real' in digital technology, becoming the only possible space for human, educational, commercial, and sharing relationships, making the futuristic dream of a digital life come true quickly and unexpectedly.

From school, public administrations, museum exhibits, archives, conferences, shows, and festivals, we realized that using the digital does not involve replacing but assisting, supporting in case of emergency, and maybe even strengthening our ability to communicate.[3] We found that another way of working is possible: working from home became the new normal, and, even if the changes came suddenly, in a very short time they consolidated ways of performing the work that had not existed before. In just a few months, a total digital transformation occurred, one that would have been years in the making.

If the COVID emergency has, in a certain way, abruptly paused our lives, it must be recognized that it has accelerated those other phenomena and processes that were first moving slowly: just think of the number of

---

3   Zhora Lassoued, Mohammed Alhendawi, Raed Bashitialshaaer, 'An Exploratory Study of the Obstacles for Achieving Quality in Distance Learning during the COVID-19 Pandemic', *Education Sciences*, 10, 2020(9), 232–45.

workers who have continued to work in a 'smart' way, the spread of digital payment systems as opposed to the poor traceability of cash money, the rapid redefinition of some companies forced to change their business in order to survive, and the amplification of connectivity that started the so-called *digital transformation*. COVID-19 has in fact disrupted all aspects of daily life, from sociality and learning to consumption and entertainment, causing major inconveniences, but also and above all, creating great opportunities.

The need to change our behavior has led us, in the most natural and immediate way, to resort to digital media that, inevitably, has impacted many aspects of our lives: the way we have social relationships has changed work, education, school, leisure, entertainment, our hobbies, the way we enjoy culture and, not least, the way we shop. We have changed the way we relate to our loved ones by using those services made available by platforms such as Skype, Teams, WhatsApp, and Zoom, just to name a few, noting that even those who were unfamiliar with these tools, such as some members from older generations, have learned to use them as well.

With the closure of schools and universities, new forms of teaching are redefining relational methods between students and teachers, as well as between teachers and families. With different timing and methods, each institution has taken action to allow for Distance Learning, including new teaching methodologies for both synchronous and asynchronous teaching.[4] Recent research by Save The Children, carried out on about 300 Italian households, found that

> Six out of ten households (57.2%) do not have a home internet connection, while almost all respondents have at least one mobile network (95.5%). It is families in southern Italy who have the most problems with home connection, of which only one in three families (33.1%), against one in two in Central Italy (51.7%) and almost one in two in Northern Italy (45.5%). Most households have two or three devices at their disposal (59.7%). More than one in ten

---

4   Asynchronous training is a training relationship situation in which the subjects communicate from different places and at different times. There is no simultaneous presence of teachers and learners, and therefore the interaction between them is obviously limited. The tools that are usually used in this training mode are different and vary between different platforms of Formation to Distance (FAD). The Massachusetts Institute of Technology (MIT) has proposed the so-called *MOOC – Massive Open Online Courses*, to reach even the population living in dispersed areas of the United States. This is an evolution of university correspondence courses that are being considered to expand for all levels of education, making them available also on television and digital platforms.

families has only one device (13.2%) and 0.3% not even that. However, the possession of a good number of devices in each family must not be misled. In fact, they are almost always smartphones, available to 98.9% of families, but less than pc, present in one in three families (30.9%) and rarely tablets, available only to one in ten families (12%).[5]

Almost a century ago, during the polio epidemic of 1937, a similar problem had to be solved in Chicago. After recording numerous cases of contagion in August, Dr. Herman Bundensen, president of the Board of Health, decided to postpone the opening of schools by three weeks. This delay started the first large-scale experiment in Distance Learning, via a highly innovative program: about 315,000 children, from 3rd to 8th grade, continued their studies from home, listening to the lessons broadcast by radio. In the late 1930s, radio was the main and most popular source of news and entertainment. More than 80% of U.S. households had at least one radio, but they were severely lacking in the South, in rural areas, and in Black households. In Chicago, teachers, under the supervision of experts in the subjects taught, took action to create lessons to be broadcasted on seven local radio stations. Through the newspapers, information was given on the timetables of the lessons of the following morning: on Mondays, Wednesdays and Fridays lessons in social studies and science were held; Tuesdays, Thursdays and Saturdays were devoted to English and mathematics. The school day was structured very simply: it began with motor activities and went into short lessons (lasting only 15 minutes each), and ended with homework assignments.

The aim was to propose a "fun" way of learning that, at the same time, could still be educational. Radio education officially ended at the end of September, when schools reopened. Although the program lasted less than three weeks, it changed the role of local Chicago radio stations: a partnership was formed between the city's public schools and its radio stations that was quickly cemented in the formation of the Chicago Radio Council. Radio shows and conferences complemented school programs and began offering students opportunities to participate in news, radio roundtables, and other educational programs.[6] Technology, therefore, has always shown itself to

---

5   Christian Morabito, *La scuola che verrà. Attese, incertezze e sogni all'avvio del nuovo anno scolastico* (Rome: Save the Children, 2020), p. 5, <https://s3. savethechildren.it/public/files/uploads/pubblicazioni/la-scuola-che-verra_0.pdf> (last access: November 15th, 2021).

6   Katherine A. Foss, *Constructing the Outbreak: Epidemics in Media and Collective Memory* (Amherst, Massachusetts: University of Massachusetts Press, 2020).

be the best tool in times of crisis, regardless of its degree of sophistication. The Chicago experiment should make us reflect not only on the importance of emergency measures in education, but we should not consider them as only temporary solutions: they could be beneficial supplements to in-person learning.

2. *The Internet effect in the time of Coronavirus*

With the aim of having a secure telecommunications network even in the event of war, the U.S. government established the ARPA (Advanced Research Project Agency) in 1958, a research center responsible for the design of a telematic network able to overcome the vulnerabilities of a centralized communication system such as the telephone. Worried that the US would lose its scientific, technological, economic, and military hegemony after the Soviets' launch of Sputnik into space, President Eisenhower formed the agency, appointing the rector of the Massachusetts Institute of Technology, James Killian, as coordinator. It was Killian's successor, engineer Lawrence Roberts, who would eventually develop the ARPANET: networks connecting dozens of systems that would permit resource sharing between thousands of users.[7]

The project officially began on December 5th, 1969, when the first four nodes of the network corresponding to four research centers in the west of the country were first connected. In 1972, the nodes rose to 25 and three years later became 60: among them was one in Hawaii, one in Norway, and another in London. By this point, the military was unable to make use of the network, so it was given to the top US universities to facilitate the dissemination of scientific information and to optimize all available computing resources: computers were not personal, they were very expensive and, of the few that existed, were the result of research projects by those same universities that shared their resources.

In 1990, ARPANET was permanently closed and the term Internet, (short for inter-networking), began to enter common language as the connections were now also open for civil use.[8] The "network of networks" was born,

---

7   Advanced Research property Project property Agency, Resource Sharing Computer Networks, Program Plan, 723 (1968), p. 1, <https://archive.org/details/ResourceSharingComputerNetworks> (last access: November 15th, 2021).

8   The American research agency that designed it, the *Advanced Research Project Agency*, began using TCP/IP transmission protocols (*Transfer Control Protocol/ Internet Protocol*) only much later, in 1983. ARPANET was the network of

and the rest is recent history. By early 2020, with the unexpected arrival of the COVID-19 virus, we saw how fundamental this network now is in keeping societies functioning and cohesive.

Thanks to the web and social networks, we have been able to reinvent daily life. Forced to stay at home as much as possible, on-demand television, multichannel, or streaming services have been far preferred over general television. News, newspapers, and news channels have mastered the response to our need to inquire, which has also guided our research on the web and on social media. One new trend was the increase in approval ratings for radio broadcasts, entertainment that was undoubtedly chosen by those who, in addition to wanting to keep a constant update on the current situation, searched for as a means to keep away the anxiety and anguish that the news itself, listing figures on the dead, the hospitalized, and the infected, transmitted at the same hours.

For the so-called creative sectors,[9] which are very much at pain from the social distancing measures adopted, massive digitalization, combined with emerging technologies such as virtual and augmented reality, have made it possible to create new forms of cultural experience and new models of dissemination of knowledge. According to a UNESCO report of May 2020, in the museum sector alone there have been almost a thousand actions in response to the COVID-19 crisis worldwide, with a large part of them aimed at promoting virtual museums, exhibitions, conferences, activities on social networks, games, educational experiences. However, the most numerous and innovative actions have been taken in the countries that have invested most in technology and have been almost absent in African states and developing states.[10]

---

academic research centers to which Italy first connected on April 30, 1986: from Pisa the first Internet signal arrived at Roaring Creek in Pennsylvania sent over the network thanks to satellites of the Telespazio center of Fucino in Abruzzo. Janet Abbate, *Inventing the Internet* (Cambridge, MA: MIT Press, 1999).

9   Land definitions of the cultural and creative sectors vary from one continent to another, but in general they cover all sectors whose activities are based on cultural values and/or artistic and creative expressions. These activities include the development, creation, production, dissemination and conservation of goods and services including architecture, archives, libraries and museums, artistic crafts, audiovisual (including film, television, video games and multimedia), material and intangible cultural heritage, design, festivals, music, literature, the performing arts, publishing, radio, visual arts, fashion.

10   UNESCO, *Museums around the world in the face of COVID-19* (Paris: UNESCO, 2020), <https://unesdoc.unesco.org/ark:/48223/pf0000373530> (last access: November 15th, 2021).

Many initiatives with a high technological content have been enhanced with the aim of allowing the vision of museum collections and artistic sites. All this has highlighted how important the use of 'cultural' content from our homes is: the *Google Arts & Culture* project, launched by Google already in 2011, perceived as an initiative aimed exclusively at art lovers, after ten years has registered a decidedly expanded target. Google's original goal was to make the digital experience additional to the material one, changing the paradigm of the use, conservation and enhancement of art and culture with innovative *machine learning technologies*.[11]

Similarly, biographical films or docufilms about the great masters of architecture, and painting, scientists, Nobel laureates, have been made available to stream on different multimedia platforms, as well as virtual tours of museums and monuments "open to the public" through digital guided tours.

Writers, bloggers and publishing houses have teamed up to launch pro-reading campaigns: online book presentations, streaming literary festivals with an interactive 'virtual audience' and laudable initiatives such as reading fragments of texts by authors to keep readers company, have intensified and today represent a 'normality'.

To mitigate the effects of lockdown, the music industry has also embraced *streaming*. To tell the truth, this phenomenon had already seen the light of day before the health emergency: in the last decade, turnover linked to the music industry had marked an important growth linked to streaming and digital downloads. Just to give an example, music-streaming platform *Spotify*, in the first quarter of 2020, registered six million subscribers, reaching a total of 130 million users.[12]

"Being connected" has also influenced the way we shop: social media has turned into real *e-commerce*[13] sites and smartphones into incredibly convenient tools to have an asset at the exact moment you feel it is needed. The so-called *conversational commerce*, voice systems 'open' to the procedures of delivery of the product in our homes have also spread to

---

11   Danilo Pesce, Paolo Neirotti, Emilio Paolucci, 'When culture meets digital platforms: value creation and stakeholders alignment in big data use', *Current Issues in Tourism*, 22(15) (2019). 1883–1903.

12   Stefan Hall, 'This is how COVID-19 is affecting the music industry', World Economic Forum, 27 May 2020, <https://www.weforum.org/agenda/2020/05/this-is-how-covid-19-is-affecting-the-music-industry/> (last access: May 30th, 2022).

13   Instagram, for example, has become a real *marketplace*: simply by following the stories of your favorite people, if they are "tagged" with products, you can buy them in real time.

which, simply giving a voice command (we ask our bear Alibaba for coffee and Starbucks delivers it to us immediately), in a short time we enjoy a delivery directly to our homes. This is a clear example of how hybridization between offline and online is increasingly rapid and immanent: change is happening on our behaviors with almost no impact on our values, almost as if there had been no choice. Digital gives us more immediate and easily achievable answers, so we adopt it almost unconsciously.

The *Weebeing* sector is also growing strongly at the moment: there are many apps useful to monitor our state of health, sleep, relaxation, meditation tools, those dedicated to nutrition, anxiety, stress and the control of disorders related to the pandemic, first and first of all depression. Silicon Valley worked hard, so much so that in a few months about ten thousand Apps have been developed (Moodpath, SuperBetter, Calm, just to mention the most downloaded), used to monitor mental health status.

In the light of these findings, it becomes inevitable to ask whether these services will be used in a non-emergency future or whether our emotional states that are triggered during the visit of a museum, at the opening of a curtain, in a literature festival or in a cinema, will make us return to our pre-pandemic habits. It is true that, just as we benefit from listening to music and watching "online" films without disdaining live concerts and cinemas, we could continue to propose a digital model to provide support to those who do not have the opportunity to travel or attend crowded places.

3. *Technostress and social distancing*

Social distancing, home isolation and remote work, although they present numerous opportunities, also lay bare certain vulnerabilities. The availability or scarcity of resources (the *comfort* of your home, the power of network connection, the quality of access devices) amplify inequalities and social distances. The pandemic has shown us these vulnerabilities; therefore, it is natural to wonder how our relationship with technology should evolve in the future.

Smart work should make the worker more productive and satisfied, but the constant monitoring of his activity certainly does not present this reality as the most desirable: digital technology makes it easier for superiors, directors and managers to contact subordinates at any time and, although there are studies that testify to an increase in productivity, a new pathology emerges, the so-called *Technostress* due precisely to having to become familiar with new technologies, face multitasking and always be available. As early as 2007, a study conducted by Ragu-Nathan and his collaborators had hypothesized the existence of five dimensions: *Overload, Invasion, Complexity, Insecurity, Uncertainty.*[14] The stereotype of the modern worker is the one that sees him in possession of at least one laptop and a corporate smartphone: the aim is to provide him with tools suitable to carry out his job even outside the office, to make it more efficient with more simultaneous tools (multitasking), as well as to put him in a position to always be available.[15] What is not considered is that the disproportionate use of digital devices only overloads the brain with information (overload), preventing the worker from resting even outside working hours and on weekends, causing him to feel invading his privacy (invasion).

Work from home often induces you to be on videoconferencing: the quality of the video call can strongly affect communication generating misunderstandings, discontent and uncertainty related to the proper functioning of the devices (uncertainty), followed by anxiety, frustration, anger, amplified also by the uncertainty related to concern for one's health, the perception that you cannot protect yourself and loved ones, the social isolation imposed by confinement.

The downside highlights that rationalization of the time leads the worker to have the opportunity to better manage his day: unnecessary hours are no longer wasted reaching the workplace or reaching places to attend meetings and give lectures. They are attended from home, perhaps combining other interactive activities.

Somehow, the futuristic dream of a digital life came true quickly and unexpectedly. What has happened must give us an indication of the possible future transformations of our societies: in the face of the surge in data traffic, the digital infrastructure has held, and this allows us to project ourselves into the future without excessive concern, but it also gives us the signal that we need to continue with investments in technology.

The difference is certainly the fragile economic situation of some households; inevitably, there is a technological gap which should not exist, especially as regards education and work activities. For example, according to OECD data, in countries such as Norway, Austria and Switzerland, 95%

---

14   Monideepa Tarafdar and others, 'The impact of technostress on role stress and productivity', *Journal of management information systems*, 24, 2007(1), 301–28.

15   Jonathan Crary photographed this situation with the expression 24/7 which indicates that you have to be active and available 24 hours a day and 7 days a week. Jonathan Crary, *24/7. Late Capitalism and the Ends of Sleep* (London-New York: To Books, 2013), pp. 8–11.

of students have a computer to use for study activities, while in Indonesia this percentage drops drastically to 34%.[16] More generally, large sections of the population in developing countries do not have the income capacity to use the technologies: for many it is impossible to buy a computer or pay for a subscription to take advantage of network connections. There is a well-founded fear that the pandemic, and the consequent increase in the use of digital systems, could accentuate the *digital divide* and its negative consequences, further reducing the possibilities for personal and professional growth. Investment and initiatives to reduce this gap must therefore be increased: the fight against digital exclusion absolutely must be launched in order to guarantee access to essential services for the digitally marginalized as well.[17]

On June 5, 1947, U.S. Secretary of State George Marshall, in a speech at Harvard, announced financial intervention by the United States in support of European countries torn apart by World War II. The European Recovery Program provided for more than $14 billion to revive the old continent's disaster economies. This funding was an extraordinary tool for Europe to transform economic, institutional and cultural structures, as well as being a source of experimentation and innovation.

In Italy, some of the funds were used to install and activate in Milan, Pisa and Rome the first electronic brains that marked the beginning of the history of computation in Italy.[18] It is hoped that the "new Marshall Plan", the so-called *Recovery Fund*, self-financed by the European Union, will once again initiate processes of economic and social transformation, allowing all European countries to invest and strengthen above all technological infrastructures in such a way as to guarantee indiscriminately networked services (health, school, justice, tourism, agriculture, electronic payments), and to strengthen those programs that expand digital skills, smart working and digital security for public administrations and businesses. It is a fine thread that combines the hopes of economic recovery of European countries, an intertwined web of innovation and sustainability, with which it is hoped that opportunities similar to those resulting from the Marshall Plan can be realized.

---

16   OECD Health Statistics 2020, <http://www.oecd.org/els/health-systems/health-data.htm> (last access: November 15th, 2021).
17   Massimo Ragnedda, *The third digital divide. A Weberian Approach to Digital Inequalities* (Rotterdam: Taylor & Francis Ltd, 2018), p. 16.
18   Carla Petrocelli, 'L'uomo che riconobbe nei numeri il futuro dell'informatica italiana', in Pietro Greco (ed. by), *Mezzogiorno di scienza. Ritratti di grandi scienziati del Sud* (Bari: Edizioni Dedalo, 2020), pp. 79–95.

4. *Limits of Artificial Intelligence*

Driven by the need to contain COVID-19, the scientific community looked to Artificial Intelligence in the hope that it could provide solutions, especially in the unawareness of the initial phase.[19] The international press, with this in mind, has taken a strong interest in the World Intelligence Congress (WIC), one of the main events dedicated to artificial intelligence held in China and which this year has been entirely reserved for issues related to the pandemic. Among the many products presented, one of the most significant was the remote temperature measurement system, proposed by Megvii and tested at Beijing metro stations to help control passengers with high fever: compared to manual measurement, the system allows you to examine up to three hundred people in one minute without interrupting the flow of passengers.[20]

In Japan, for example, robots are being perfected that can interact with the elderly to keep them company and thus avoid total isolation. Then there is an Italian project that uses predictive data, with which it's possible to define how and when to intervene on the sick to prevent them from getting worse.[21]

Regarding the search for an effective vaccine or medical treatment, AI has been used to accelerate genome sequencing, make faster diagnoses, perform scanner analysis or, more occasionally, use maintenance and delivery robots. The American startup Moderna has distinguished itself for the use of biotechnology based on messenger ribonucleic acid (mRNA) with which it has managed to significantly reduce the time it takes to develop a prototype vaccine that can be tested on humans.

The giants IBM, Amazon, Google and Microsoft have also raised awareness making available the computing power of their servers to the US authorities for processing datasets in epidemiology, bioinformatics and molecular modeling. The tools of AI have also been used to analyze

---

19 David Yakobovitch, 'How to Fight the Coronavirus with AI and Data Science', Medium, 15 February 2020, <https://towardsdatascience.com/how-to-fight-the-coronavirus-with-ai-and-data-science-b3b701f8a08a> (last access: November 15th, 2021).

20 Andy Hon Way Chun, 'In a time of coronavirus, Chinas investment in AI is paying off in a big way', South China Morning Post, 18 March 2020, <https://www.scmp.com/comment/opinion/article/3075553/time-coronavirus-chinas-investment-ai-paying-big-way> (last access: November 15th, 2021).

21 Gabriel A. Brat and others, 'International Electronic Health Record-Derived COVID-19 Clinical Course Profile: The 4CE Consortium', *Digital Medicine*, 3, 109 (2020), <https://doi.org/10.1038/s41746-020-00308-0> (last access: November 15th, 2021).

the thousands of research papers published worldwide on the pandemic: the massive production of scientific literature represents a real challenge for anyone hoping to analyze, in their entirety, the research. Predictive modelling has made progress, thanks to new data sources and computational techniques, and has greatly improved over the last decade: one model serves primarily to reason about scenarios, simulate them, and understand what might or might not work by leaning in favor of one choice over another. The real impact of data science would be to be able to create policies to tackle the problem before the problem becomes worse.[22]

Data modelling, crowds screening and contact tracking were therefore the main lines of research on which work has been done in this area. In fact, the role of Artificial Intelligence in recent months has seemed far from central and even the hopes placed in *contact tracing systems* have not been satisfactory. In the European context, we have seen a first attempt to establish common standards which has been somewhat diminished by national differences on data collection and processing. This has provoked a real questioning of the technological tool in the context of the COVID-19 crisis, which has also led to the hypothesis of its non-use in those countries where political contraindications have been manifested.

More useful, perhaps, was the use of artificial intelligence-based filters, activated by social media managers to counter the phenomenon of *fake news*. AI is indeed proven to be a sufficiently effective technology to control inappropriate content posted on social platforms, also following UNICEF directives that in providing information about the virus, government authorities and online partners such as Facebook, Instagram, LinkedIn and TikTok, should take measures to inform the public when inaccurate information appears.[23]

5. The world to come

The COVID-19 crisis has shown how important technology can be in times of change and uncertainty. When will we resume our pre–covid-19

---

22 Bani Sapra, 'Googles DeepMind just shared AI-generated predictions about the coronavirus that could help researchers stem the global outbreak', Business Insider, 5 March 2020, <https://www.businessinsider.com/google-deepmind-ai-predictions-coronavirus-2020-3> (last access: November 15th, 2021).

23 Statement from Charlotte Petri Gornitzka, UNICEF Deputy Executive Director for Partnerships, <https://www.unicef.it/media/unicef-stop-a-disinformazione-e-fake-news-sul-coronavirus/> (last access: November 15th, 2021).

life, access to these services will be reduced, but some habits will remain: the psychological obstacle of their use has certainly been overcome, even if forcibly. The isolation to which the global pandemic has forced us has meant that 'being connected' is no longer perceived as something additional, but as a substantial moment in our lives as citizens, consumers and workers: with the use of technology for access to basic services such as health and education, fair management of the digital divide becomes of primary importance, in order to ensure social equality.

In a few weeks we have witnessed a real transfer to the network of economic, work, relational and educational activities and the futuristic dream of a digital life has come true quickly and unexpectedly. The COVID-19 crisis has shed light on the great territorial inequalities in access to the Internet and Information and Communications Technology (ICT)[24]: OECD data show that the differences in household access to broadband are significant, with important variations between individual countries.[25] What has happened must give the right indication of the way forward in the future transformations of our societies. In the face of soaring data traffic, digital infrastructure has held up. However, we will have to project ourselves into tomorrow, encouraging the investments necessary to connect the whole territory, also looking carefully at the use of energy that should rely on renewable sources and have eco-sustainability objectives.

In order to avoid passively managing this transformation, reference should be made to a plan that can be shared at European, if not global, level, a "Digital Agenda" that tackles the main stumbling block represented by the digital divide. It is clear, by the very nature of technological innovation, that governance will only be effective if it is a moment of dialogue and comparison between the different competences provided by science, philosophy and any other form of human knowledge implicit in the phenomena described. The various actors involved need to be engaged in a constructive and coordinated logic: the institutional world, academia and technology companies should reflect on the steps to be taken towards an efficient use of technology to fully realize the opportunities offered.[26]

---

24   The set of methods and techniques used in the transmission, reception and processing of data and information.

25   OECD Regional Statistics (database): <https://www.oecd.org/digital/broadband-statistics-update.htm> (last access: November 15th, 2021).

26   The *Governance* it is the space where anthropological and ethical considerations, in mutual exchange and dialogue, must become effective forces to shape and guide the technological innovation, making it an authentic source of human development. Pietro Lacorte, Giovanni Scarafile, Renato Balduzzi (eds.), *La*

Technology can give us countless benefits to which, surely, we will no longer be able to give up and, indeed we will take them more and more for granted as if they were our right, an additional "arm" at our disposal. The difference between digital and real will therefore be less and less relevant: in presence or remotely, with e-commerce or in-store, online or offline, we will choose from time to time what will seem most convenient to us.

In the 1950s, when computers occupied entire rooms, humans walked between their parts; the technology then transformed these electronic pachyderms into personal devices that, with the addition of touch screens, icons, apps, listening devices, voice commands, Siri, Alexa, Google Maps have become wearable. With this additional potential derived from connections, machines, as a tool to explore the world, have become "our" world.

The lockdown represented a period of collective learning on the role of data in society and accelerated the emergence or spread of activism practices around this data: social relationships, personal life, work, shopping, school, leisure, hobbies, are therefore profoundly changed and probably also permanently.

These collective and individual changes are certainly not easy. It may well be that we humans will not be able to improve our standards, even after these tragic events. Evolution will take its course. Darwin, prophetically, explained it well:

As many more individuals of each species are born than can possibly survive; and as, consequently, there is a frequently recurring struggle for existence, it follows that any being, if it vary however slightly in any manner profitable to itself, under the complex and sometimes varying conditions of life, will have a better chance of surviving, and thus be naturally selected.[27]

---

governance dello sviluppo: etica, economia, politica, scienza (Rome: Ave, 2004), p. 43.

27   Charles R. Darwin, *On the origin of species by means of natural selection, or the preservation of favored races in the struggle for life* (London: John Murray, 1859), p. 5.

GUIDO BAGGIO

HABITS BETWEEN VIRUS AND STATE OF EXCEPTION

1. COVID and the state of exception. A brief history of the popularization of a dogma

During the first lockdown period, the political restrictions on activities, travel and social gatherings provoked philosophers and intellectuals to reflect on the relationship between political power and individual liberty. The debate can be traced back to Giorgio Agamben's intervention on February 27th (2020), *L'invenzione di una pandemia* [*The invention of a pandemic*]. In this contribution, Agamben criticised the government for having adopted "frenetic, irrational and completely unjustified" emergency measures on the basis of a supposed pandemic. He pointed to these measures and the spread of panic by the media and authorities as the expression of "a real state of exception, with serious restrictions on movement and a suspension of the normal functioning of living and working conditions in entire regions". He then argued that the 'invention' of the pandemic was a way of maintaining a perpetual state of fear that kept growing in people's minds. "Thus, in a perverse vicious circle, the limitation of freedom imposed by governments is accepted in the name of a desire for security that has been induced by the same governments that now intervene to satisfy it".[1] To sum up his view, the 'alleged' state of emergency was just a way to support "the growing tendency to use the state of exception as the normal paradigm of government".[2]

For a better understanding of Agamben's critique, it is necessary to draw attention to his discussion of the 'state of exception', a key concept he has developed since the 1990s within his theoretical-political

---

1   Giorgio Agamben, 'L'invenzione di una pandemia', *Una voce*, 26 February, 2020 <https://www.quodlibet.it/giorgio-agamben-l-invenzione-di-un-epidemia>, my translation (last access: November 13th, 2021).
2   See: Giorgio Agamben, *Stato di eccezione* (Turin: Bollati Boringhieri, 2003) [engl. tr. *State of Exception*, (Chicago: Chicago University Press, 2005)].

paradigm. The notion of 'state of exception', as used in the legal and political spheres, denotes a suspension of the constitutional order — or at least a significant part of it — by the same state authority that should normally be the guarantee of legality. While remaining within the legal sphere of the rule of law, this suspension is expressed in the collapse of the equilibrium existing between 'norm' and 'decision', resulting in the complete autonomisation of the latter. Instead of the norm, the sovereign power produces other acts — decrees and regulations issued by the government — which, while anomic, have legal force and are imposed with the same effectiveness as the norm. The dialectical relationship between the normative element and the anomic element can be traced back to the dialectical relationship between *potestas* and *auctoritas*, according to which "the normative element [*potestas*] needs the anomic element in order to apply itself, but, on the other hand, the *auctoritas* can only affirm itself in a relationship of validation or suspension of the *potestas*".[3] With the state of exception, *potestas* and *auctoritas* coincide in the same subject of power, which conveys within itself both the instituting and the destituent power. The state of exception thus reveals itself as a legal *a-topos*, a space of anomie from which, however, emanates an essential force for the legal system itself. In fact, the latter could not even exist if it were not based on a sovereign decision involving the transformation of a previous order or its destruction in the extreme. According to Agamben, the 'state of exception' has become commonplace in the context of Western capitalist democracies to the detriment of a state of law and its ability to limit the violence of a government power which "nevertheless claims to still be applying the law".[4] In his essay on the state of exception, Agamben had already noted that in the Italian political context, since the first unification, the use of decree-law as an ordinary source of legislation marked the transition of 'parliamentary democracy' into 'governmental democracy'. In his most recent tirade against Italian government measures, he therefore reiterates the systematic and regular use of ministerial decrees which, in the long run, undermines democracy and the legislative function of Parliament. The latter indeed is increasingly relegated to a mere ratifier of government measures.

Several philosophers and intellectuals have objected Agamben's intervention. Jean-Luc Nancy, for instance, criticised Agamben for missing the target, arguing that blaming governments was "more like a

---

3   Agamben, *Stato di eccezione*, pp. 109-10 [engl. tr., p. 86].
4   *Ibid.*, p. 111 [engl. tr., p. 87].

diversionary manoeuvre than a political reflection".[5] Roberto Esposito, on the other hand, accused Agamben of having ignored "the historically differentiated character of biopolitical phenomena" and of losing "his sense of proportion".[6]

It should be noted that in the initial phases of the pandemic, Agamben's criticism relied on the advice of the Italian National Research Center (CNR) and other international research organisations, including the World Health Organization (WHO), which downplayed the severity of the virus. Unfortunately, only a few days later, the health situation turned out to be increasingly serious at the national and global levels. As a result, even if in a disordered way, the international scientific and medical community corrected its opinion on a phenomenon whose behaviour was proving to be more obscure, unforeseeable and aggressive than expected. Within this changing scenario, however, Agamben maintained his position, mainly reiterating the paradigm of the state of exception to describe the current pandemic situation. Deepening his reflections in a second intervention on the 'hunting of unctors', which took its cue from the restrictions on people who would exercise physical activity outdoors, and in a *Chiarimento* [*Clarification*] (March 17th), he essentially reiterated the paradigm of the state of exception as the key to interpret the current pandemic situation:

> The bare life — and the fear of losing it — is not something that unites people, but blinds and separates them. Other human beings, as in the plague described by Manzoni, are now seen only as possible unctors that must be avoided at all costs and from whom one must keep at least a meter's distance. People who died – our people – do not have the right to a funeral and it is not clear what happens to the bodies of our loved ones. Our neighbor has been removed and it is astonishing that churches are silent on the matter. What do human relationships become in a country that gets used to living this way for no one knows how long? And what is a society that has no value other than survival?[7]

5   Jean-Luc Nancy, 'Eccezione virale', *Antinomie. Scritture e immagini*, 27 February, 2020 <https://antinomie.it/index.php/2020/02/27/eccezione-virale/>, my translation (last access: November 13th, 2021).

6   Roberto Esposito, 'Curati a oltranza', *Antinomie. Scritture e immagini*, 27 February, 2020 <https://antinomie.it/index.php/2020/02/28/curati-a-oltranza/>, my translation (last access: November 13th, 2021).

7   Giorgio Agamben, 'Chiarimenti', *Una voce*, 17 March 2020 <https://www.quodlibet.it/giorgio-agamben-chiarimenti>, my translation (last access: November 13th, 2021).

Referring to the other key concept of his paradigm, 'bare life', Agamben drew precisely on the fear of the virus, proof of a process that shifted our priorities from the centrality of human, emotional, social, and political life to the inalienability of biological life. He therefore warned us that a society which, living in a perpetual state of emergency primarily for security, cannot be a free society but a tyrannical one, since it condemns us to live in a perpetual state of fear and insecurity.

Agamben's dystopian–Orwellian projection of such a state of exception envisaged the disappearance of universities and schools, replaced by online lectures, as well as the disappearance of opportunities and places for political and cultural aggregation and eventually the replacement of all contact between human beings by machines. In other words, he was indicating a change in mental and behavioural habits that could only be catastrophic.[8]

2. *Scientific belief and dogmatic truth*

In line with the denialist trend, in the following intervention, *Riflessioni sulla peste* [*Reflections on the plague*] (March 27th), Agamben questioned the importance of science, which in his view has grown to the point of satisfying those religious needs of individuals that the Church is no longer able to meet. Only one month after he referred to the national and international scientific institutions (CNR and WHO) to support his idea that

---

8   Mario Farina, among others, criticised Agamben's tendentious and rhetorical translation of Benjamin's '*bloße Leben*' and likened Agamben's invective against government restrictions to the public dances of Bolsonaro's supporters against the international pandemic conspiracy and to the first positions taken by Donald Trump and Boris Johnson, who thought it more important to save economic production, and therefore social relations, rather than life and public welfare. See: Mario Farina, 'Su Agamben e il contagio. Il ruolo della filosofia e la comune umanità', *Le parole e le cose*, 20 March 2020 <http://www.leparoleelecose. it/?p=37978> (last access: November 13th, 2021). Luca Illetterati, on the other hand, questioned the Agambenian theoretical proposal that reduces individual life to a mere product of the device of power, which would have as its sole objective the control of lives and their actions. In particular, Illetterati criticized Agamben's assumption of the difference between 'bare life' on the one hand, and life in its fullest sense, i.e. as affective, social and political life, on the other. He argues that this distinction, instead of overcoming certain abstractions and presuppositions, assumes them as decisive. (Luca Illetterati, 'Dal contagio alla vita. E ritorno. Ancora in margine alle parole di Agamben', *Le parole e le cose*, 31 March 2020 <http://www.leparoleelecose.it/?p=38033> (last access: November 13th, 2021).

the government invented the pandemic to corroborate a state of exception, Agamben contradicted himself by claiming that science "can produce superstition and fear or, in any case, be used to spread them" through a spectacularization in public debates of the contradictory opinions and the prescriptions of scientists.[9] When doubts arise about the current situation, talk-shows get crowded with supporters of opposing factions who make its contrasts more radical. This strategy leads people to think that the political power's preference for the opinions of scientists is not so much the result of an attribution of epistemic dignity to their knowledge – an attribution grounded in concrete evidence and dialectical interpretations – but rather the expression of a power which, "as at the time of the religious disputes takes sides according to its own interests for one current or another and imposes its measures".[10] The state of exception paradigm thus shifts to the instrumental role that scientific knowledge plays in legitimising political power.

Now, Agamben's critique of scientific knowledge relies on a questionable inference made from scientific belief to the religious role that scientific knowledge plays in our society today. This inference seems to develop as follows: if the science on which the system of restrictions on our liberty stands does not possess definite truths about the virus, then any use of scientific belief to restrict liberty is as despotic and dogmatic as religion has been in the past.

As I will briefly state, this tricky inference stems from what Charles Sanders Peirce would have called a 'habit of mind', that is, a way of drawing a particular inference from certain pre-constituted premises based on some kind of belief. This habit of mind, which reflects a widespread attitude today equating scientific rhetoric with political rhetoric, is the ultimate expression of a process of change that has been going on in science and which has resulted in the transformation of scientific questions into linguistic ones.

To illustrate how this tricky inference is made from the uncertainty of science to the despotic dogmatism of anomic power, I would recall the distinction made by Peirce between behaviour guided by beliefs imposed by an authority and behaviour guided by beliefs based on the scientific

---

9   Giorgio Agamben, 'Riflessioni sulla peste', *Una voce*, 27 March 2020 <https://www.quodlibet.it/giorgio-agamben-riflessioni-sulla-peste>, my translation (last access: November 13th, 2021).

10   Agamben, 'Riflessioni sulla peste'.

method.[11] According to the authority method, a state imposes beliefs on its citizens that are judged to be correct, coercively preventing the affirmation, expression or dissemination of conflicting beliefs. Dogmatism, in this case, is based on a despotic will to subjugate individuals and expresses itself in an absolute arbitrariness on the part of authority over the individual's choices. The uniformity of opinions is ensured by "a moral terrorism to which the respectability of society will give its thorough approval".[12] Applying Peirce's description to the current state of emergency, one could say that the power of government is the way to public health, and that the plea for individual responsibility is the moral terrorism to which the 'respectable society', which accepts restrictions, gives its full approval by constructing a uniform opinion on the need to respect the rules. Although this method is typical of a theocratic or dictatorial state, it would seem that, in the case of a pandemic emergency such as the present one, it is also used in democratic states. If this were the case, one could agree with Agamben's observation about the ease with which an entire society accepts to feel afflicted, to isolate itself at home, and to suspend its normal living conditions.[13]

However, the authority method shows a great limitation, especially when it is exercised in democratic societies that guarantee liberty of thought and expression: the limitation concerns the social feeling of dissent that questions the convictions proposed by the authorities, raising questions and doubts about the validity of these convictions and therefore the legitimacy of the restrictions. In this respect, the very possibility of criticising government choices, of being able to oppose opinions, is an expression of this non-conformity to the system. In other words, the manifestation of non-conformity sheds a doubt at least "upon every proposition which is considered essential to the security [or health] of society".[14] It is precisely this shadow of doubt that hangs over the actions of governments and allows us to measure the degree of opportunism of political choices in a state of emergency and the risk of an authoritarian deviation. The role of intellectuals such as Agamben is precisely to highlight the risk of such a deviation. As Agamben has repeatedly stressed in recent months, basing

---

11   See: Charles S. Peirce, 'The Fixation of Belief', *Popular Science Monthly*, 12 (1877), pp. 1–15; republished in *Writing of Charles Sanders Peirce*, edited by Peirce Edition Project (Indianapolis and Bloomington: Indiana University Press, 1981–2000), vol. III [W3.243–57].

12   Peirce, W3.255.

13   See: Agamben, 'Riflessioni sulla peste'.

14   Peirce, W3.256.

the authority of power on the fear of losing one's life can only lead to legitimising tyranny and not a democratic and liberal society.

Even more, as opposed to the method of purely dogmatic authority, in a state of emergency such as the one we are experiencing, the legitimacy of democratic decision-making authority is rooted in the presumed validity of the scientific belief that there is a *real* phenomenon — the virus — that poses a threat to public health.[15] In other words, the method of authority seems to be limited and legitimised by the other method set out by Peirce, namely the scientific method.

The validation of the state of emergency is in fact expressed in the prescriptive statements of the political power — 'it is compulsory to wear a mask when outdoors'; 'it is forbidden to go out of the house from 10 p.m. to 5 a.m.'; etc. — relying on the denotative statements of science — i.e. 'the virus is spread by coughing and sneezing'; 'those over 70 years of age and with pre-existing conditions are more likely to develop severe forms of illness', etc.

According to the scientific method, the formation of shared beliefs is based on the search for some uniformity that can be found in reality, and involves a research community that validates facts through their interpretation. In other words, scientific research is like a three-legged stool, where one leg is the subjective (the scientist), one is the objective reality (the phenomenon studied), and the third is the intersubjective comparison (the scientific community).[16] Without any of these three legs the stool does not stand. Thus, the contrast between different opinions within the scientific community, where uniformity is still far from being achieved on many points — as seems to be the case with COVID-19

---

15 Peirce, W3.253: "Such is the method of science. Its fundamental hypothesis, restated in more familiar language, is this: There are Real things, whose characters are entirely independent of our opinions about them; those Reals affect our senses according to regular laws, and, though our sensations are as different as are our relations to the objects, yet, by taking advantage of the laws of perception, we can ascertain by reasoning how things really and truly are; and any man, if he have sufficient experience and he reason enough about it, will be led to the one True conclusion."

16 The reference to the three-legged stool is drawn from Hilary Putnam's idea of the intertwining of facts, theories and values in scientific research but is interpreted here in a more Davidsonian way. Cf. Hilary Putnam, *The collapse of the fact/value dichotomy and other essays* (Cambridge: Harvard University Press, 2002); 'Hilary Putnam interviewed by Naoko Saito and Paul Standish', *Journal of Philosophy of Education*, vol. 48, 1 (2014), p. 24; D. Davidson, *Subjective, Intersubjective, Objective* (Oxford: Clarendon Press, 2001).

— shows that scientific truth is not dogmatic and authoritarian, but rather collegial and in the making. It is based on the comparison between different interpretations of the data collected and takes place in a community that assumes doubt and fallibility as guiding principles of research. The difficulty of reaching a consensus, particularly if the phenomenon investigated is relatively new, lies at the heart of scientific enquiry and its ordinary research processes. In this respect, within the scientific community the dialectic among experts is essential to the process of enquiry.

Difficulties arise when members of the scientific community are consulted by the wider non-expert community. In this case, scientific dialectic could be understood by the wider community of non-experts, but also, as is the case of Agamben, by philosophers, as the only element that can decide the validity of a scientific opinion. In fact, if the scientific community itself does not yet have a shared opinion, among the different ways of expressing dissent the most detrimental to the credibility of the scientific community is the one we often witness in public debates, in which experts disagree among themselves, even offending each other in public, 'as politicians do'. In such cases, the non-experts watching this unfortunate show and, at the same time, having to follow the restricting rules decreed by those same scientists offending each other there on live TV, interpret disagreement between scientists not so much as the confrontation between different perspectives, but as the expression of sectarian disputes. Rigorists versus tolerants, alarmists versus negationists, discuss their respective scientific positions in public arenas, which are very unsuitable places for specialised debates and much more appropriate for feeding the vanity of individuals. The result of this distortion is the polarisation of public opinion between disaffection with scientific knowledge and its dogmatisation, which can be easily misused in political disputes.

Now, despite the fact that many possible hypotheses on the genesis of this clash can be formulated, I would propose to use Lyotard's discussion on the condition of knowledge in postmodern society, to argue that the assimilation of *scientific rhetoric* into *political rhetoric* is the ultimate expression of a changing process of knowledge which began in the second half of the nineteenth century. This process, which turned *scientific issues* into *linguistic issues*, is strictly intertwined with the computerisation and simplification of knowledge that has characterised post-industrial societies since the post-Second World War and which exasperates the productive character of language to the detriment of an increasingly problematic adherence to truth and factual reality.[17] It is tied also to (or 'it involves also') the progressive assimilation of scientific dialectics to political polemics, in the deterrent sense of the concept of *pólemos* that we are witnessing today and which stresses the role of the paralogical capacity of language in re-describing, re-interpreting, and constructing continuous disagreements with the existing descriptions of a given phenomenon.[18] On this view, scientific, i.e. denotative statements are legitimised as true by a linguistic dispute where denotative statements are supported by rhetorical statements. In other words, persuasion, which agonistically opposes the arguments of contrasting positions, falls within the realm of *scientific pragmatics*.

If scientific disputes with their rhetorical statements are performed in front of a non-expert audience, doubts, dissents, and falsifications — all elements belonging to the process of scientific enquiry — can easily be misunderstood. And this misunderstanding produces in non-experts the same scepticism that surrounds political debates, where the real goal is the search for electoral consensus and not the search for a shared vision. In short, there is a flattening of the *episteme* into the *doxa*. The scientific community's debate is effectively absorbed into the political debate, so that the legitimisation or delegitimisation of its value is achieved through a distortion of the rhetorical process of the scientific community.[19] It is precisely from this distortion, and the resulting confusion between the scientific and political levels of discourse, that the problematic interplay between scientific and political credibility emerges. Traditional problematic issues related to the confusion between power and knowledge emerge explicitly, such as the question of who has the power to decide what is scientifically true and what is politically correct. This goes back to the essential question concerning the autonomy of

---

17 As early as 1979, Jean-François Lyotard outlined in his pamphlet *The Postmodern Condition: A Report on Knowledge* (Minneapolis: University of Minneapolis Press, 1984) a cartography of the condition of knowledge in post-industrial western society. He highlighted the increasing centrality of language, as well as the revision of paradigms and modes of reasoning in the sciences, as the causes of the change in the status of knowledge from an instrument of social emancipation to an element dependent on technological informatization. On post-truth see Giovanni Maddalena, Guido Gili, *The History and Theory of Post-Truth Communication* (London: Palgrave Macmillan, 2020).

18 On the positive meaning of conflict see: Umberto Curi, *Pólemos. Filosofia come guerra* (Turin: Bollati Boringhieri, 2000).

19 As well as the work of Lyotard, Habermas' reflections on the legitimacy of scientific knowledge are still relevant. Cf. Jürgen Habermas, *Knowledge and Human Interests* (Boston: Polity Press, 1987).

scientific research from political and economic power. In the specific case of the state of emergency, the conflation between the legitimation of scientific truth and the legitimation of political power results in theoretical-political interpretations which, by denouncing the anomalous nature of the exercise of political power, go so far as to delegitimise the scientific knowledge associated with it.[20] Dissent among scientists is thus used to challenge political choices, arguing that since there is no shared consensus, the position taken by the institutions could express the political interest in enslaving the population to governmental choices through an authoritarian approach. In this context, the decision to restrict individual freedoms can be interpreted as arbitrary.[21] The suspicion here is justified by the fact that certain scientific beliefs are interpreted as dogmatic by politics and uniformity is ensured through moral terrorism to which society gives its approval.

However, this conflation between the legitimation of scientific truth and the legitimation of political power highlights a greater risk: it can lead to controversial (and popular) interpretations such as that of Agamben & other 'heretic warriors' like Enrico Montesano.[22]

3. *Dissenting and disobeying*

As we have seen, Agamben believes that science has assumed the role that religion once had of appeasing uncertainty and fear. This role attributed to science rests on truths that risk becoming dogmatic: although scientific beliefs are being constructed and are a source of dialectic within the scientific community itself, this dialectic can be misused by political power. This means that the exercise of governmental power in a state of emergency in choosing which scientific interpretation to accept risks an authoritarian deviation that undermines the inalienable freedoms of citizens. It is then legitimate and desirable, according to Agamben, to express dissent and disobey the rules. It is grafted onto the more general question of civil responsibility.

---

20 On the legitimacy of the authority of international organizations see Jonas Tallberg, Michael Zürn, 'The legitimacy and legitimation of international organizations: introduction and framework', *The Review of International Organizations*, 14 (2019), 581–606.

21 Cfr. Jean-François Lyotard, *Le postmoderne expliqué aux enfants* (Paris: Galilée, 2005), pp. 93–4.

22 Enrico Montesano, *Pochi eretici guerrieri* <https://www.youtube.com/watch?v=ochChSDgyrg> (last access: November 13th, 2021).

Given Agamben's position, I would like to try to shift the perspective from which to look at the issue, departing slightly from the level of the relationship between coercion of individual freedom and disobedience. If responsibility is the tool that we as citizens of constitutional democracies have and that the rules assume, whether they are enacted in a situation of normal administration or in a state of emergency, then, it seems to me that in the specific pandemic context that we are experiencing, the rhetoric of disobedience does not contribute significantly to raise awareness of individual responsibility on a political level. Rather, it is an expression of a refractory attitude towards accepting the inescapable adherence to the contingency of reality, showing itself to be ultimately prey to a dogmatism of rivalry.

In particular, COVID-19 has highlighted the limits of an individualistic and abstract idea of liberty as well as of a minimal conception of responsibility on which the aforementioned association between silence and obedience and its counterpart is rooted. In fact, the appeal to individual responsibility, in addition to highlighting the limits of institutions, reveals the limit of an idea of freedom that is implicitly accepted in all critical discussions that oppose the state of exception and emergency sovereignty. This conception of freedom is rooted in a modern idea of the human being whereby the possibilities of choice are characterised as logical possibilities offered to a foolish mind that can choose in the absoluteness of all possibilities, without having to come to terms with the concrete conditions of the socio-historical context.[23]

The pandemic highlighted that while the free expression of scepticism and dissent against a policy of fear based on threat as a control mechanism and the denunciation of the irresponsibility of institutions with respect to the weight of responsibility they delegate to us citizens is fundamental for assessing the health of a democracy, disobedience to the rules is not necessarily the best way to manifest such dissent. In short, the reference to responsibility, be it individual, collective, or institutional, highlights the need to pay attention to the context in which it is exercised, so as to make it possible to put every issue of theoretical, political, and social criticism to the test of everyday life. Therefore, to Agamben's accusation that we Italians are willing to sacrifice practically everything, from normal living conditions, social relations, and work, to friendships, affections, and even religious and political convictions in order to safeguard '*bloße Leben*', one

---

23   See: Francesco Valerio Tommasi, 'Curarsi di. Una libertà inchiodata al corpo e alla storia', *Le parole e le cose*, 14 April, 2020 <http://www.leparoleelecose. it/?p=38132> (last access: November 13th, 2021).

could counter with Mario Farina that this accusation does not take into account that the 'practically everything' we sacrifice is done not only to safeguard our own lives but also to protect the lives of others, and that the very wellbeing we seek to safeguard for our own bodies is the essential and inalienable basis on which the common humanity is built, which, universalised, can be the sole source of equality between human beings.[24]

On a more abstract and general level of reflection, however, one might note that within the broader framework of discussion on the relationship between *auctoritas* and *potestas* on which the state of exception is grafted, even the act of disobedience to the law represents the expression of the state of exception, that is, of the disjunction of the legal norm from its application (or force of law),[25] and therefore contributes as much as the exercise of power to generating an anomic space.

4. *A very brief conclusion*

If, according to Agamben, the production of the 'effective state of exception' is a necessary test case for cutting the link between violence and law and responding to the planetary deployment of the state of exception that accompanies the globalisation of capital, he nevertheless fails to consider the contingency of the reality that today's pandemic represents. On the strength of a general theoretical paradigm through which to read the events of human political existence, Agamben continues to look for contingent signs that confirm the perpetuation of the state of exception and the limitation of individual freedoms as the fruit of a cumbersome system of capitalist power. Of course, as is well known, if we already know what we are looking for, the work of validation is much easier and perhaps even obvious. It would perhaps be interesting if Agamben were to look for elements that falsify his theory.

---

24   Farina, 'Su Agamben e il contagio'.
25   Roberto Simoncini, 'Un concetto di diritto pubblico: lo 'stato di eccezione' secondo Giorgio Agamben', *Diritto e questioni pubbliche*, 8 (2008), p. 210.

Catherine Dromelet

UNSUSTAINABLE HEALTHY HABITS
Pandemic Restrictions against the Background of Durkheim's Theory of Rituals

Introduction

Considering the events related to the pandemic, one easily observes that the restrictive measures that have been implemented in most countries in order to contain the virus spread have represented a drastic change in people's habits. With all its practical implications, this multifaceted change undeniably arouses negative feelings, widely ranging from frustration to despair. It is not an overstatement to talk about one of the main effects of the pandemic on people in terms of global panic.

In the following pages I propose to interpret the panic resulting from pandemic restrictions through the lens of classical sociologists, who can be considered as part of a tradition rooted in Durkheim's works.[1] Despite habit not being a core concept in his social theory, Durkheim still provides fruitful insights in *The Elementary Forms of Religious Life* (1912) and in other writings on morality and society. By way of introduction and based on these texts, I will start with a brief reconstruction of the way habits gather people around rituals, which determine the identity of the social group, and endow it with a sacrosanct nature.

According to Durkheim, habit is a principle that preserves the past in the present.[2] In practical terms, it allows children to internalize pre-existing social codes and learn discipline. It also enables them to emancipate, to a certain extent, from the social class where they were born. Social

---

1   Philip Smith, *Durkheim and After. The Durkheimian Tradition, 1893–2020* (Cambridge, Medford MA: Polity, 2020); Jonathan S. Fish, *Defending the Durkheimian Tradition: Religion, Emotion and Morality* (London and New York: Routledge, 2016, 2nd edn.)

2   Émile Durkheim, 'L'habitude' (lecture 34), *Cours de philosophie fait au Lycée de Sens: sections A et B, 1884* (electronic ed. by Daniel Banda and Jean-Marie Tremblay, Québec, 2002), 163–67. On the concept of habit in Durkheim, see also Marco Piazza, *Creature dell'abitudine, Abito, costume, seconda natura da Aristotele alle scienze cognitive* (Bologna: Il Mulino, 2018), pp. 212–15.

emancipation consists for an individual in developing certain habits whose acquisition is not dependent on their origins or congenital constitution.[3] However on the level of the community, shared habits is perhaps most importantly what stabilizes specific social functions, establishing customs susceptible to crystallizing, eventually, as policy-making institutions. In this view, the rigid institutional aspects of human societies ultimately result from originally a-rational, changeable underpinning dynamics, such as habits and mores.

> Each province, each territorial division, has its peculiar customs and manners, a life peculiar unto itself. It therefore exercises over the individuals who are affected by it[,] an attraction which tends to keep itself alive, and to repel all opposing forces.[4]

Customs are inclusive, in so far as they generate attraction between people engaging in them. But, since they revolve around worshipped values and 'repel all opposing forces', they are also exclusive. Inclusion allows the group to exist, while exclusion determines the group identity in opposition to other groups and their antagonist beliefs. The celebration of common values in the group is performed through a set of practices that Durkheim calls "rituals". In *The Elementary Forms of Religious Life* Durkheim develops extensively on the topic of rituals, both in religious and secular contexts. Simply put, a ritual is a collective customary practice that refers to a sacred object and is performed according to specific rules. Although sacredness is usually thought of as a characteristic peculiar to religious objects of cult, Durkheim overcomes this condition by putting forward an interesting equation between God and society: he suggests indeed that the symbolic power of society over humans is actually what the idea of god stands for: "Is it not [that] the god and the society are one and the same? [...] Society in general, simply by its effect on men's minds, undoubtedly has all that is required to arouse the sensation of the divine".[5]

As society falls within the divine, sacredness is broadened to include both secular and religious objects of worship. Any collective practice celebrating values that are essential to the identity of society can therefore be interpreted as a ritual.

---

3   Émile Durkheim, *On Morality and Society; Selected Writings*, Robert N. Bellah ed., (Chiacago: The University of Chicago Press, 1973), pp. 115–16.
4   Durkheim, p. 74.
5   Émile Durkheim, *The Elementary Forms of Religious Life*, trans. by Karen E. Fields (New York: The Free Press, 1995), p. 208.

In the following pages I start by stressing Durkheim's distinction between community and society on the basis of *The Division of Labour in Society* (1893). In this respect, Hans Joas' use of Durkheim's theory of rituals (2011) provides a useful framework to understand the process of sacralisation of the person, taking place in modern society and giving rise to individualism. However, Collins's social theory (1982) will be resorted to in order to clarify the ambivalent relationship between individuals and modern society. This tense relationship is also salient in Goffman's theory of the self as performer (1956) — a theory developed on Durkheimian premises concerning the sacredness of the person. The second section thus addresses the rituals of self-sacralisation that commonly used to take place in modern societies before the virus outbreak. The third section outlines some obstacles littering people's way to perform sacralising rituals under pandemic restrictions, resulting in a safety paradox. The ins and outs of this paradox will be interpreted in terms of a breach within social solidarity, where social organs interfere with deeply rooted habits that pertain to mechanical solidarity. In conclusion I will hint at possible consequences of our new 'healthy' pandemic habits, especially when it comes to self-esteem regulation, considering our massive reliance on communication technologies and social media as a way to compensate for social distancing.

1. *The sacralisation of the person*

While rituals act as a gravitational force keeping the community united, they are not sufficient to foster its expansion and turn it into a fully-fledged modern society. Communities or traditional societies are characterized by social similarities, which Durkheim also refers to as "mechanical solidarity";[6] it designates a model of social interactions in which crime is counter-balanced by repressive, penal law. It takes the emergence of social organs such as institutions to give rise to modern "organic solidarity",[7] where the establishment of restitutive law represents a different type of sanction for crime — namely, the payment of damages and interest. In this setting people are no longer merely interacting with one another or being subject to direct retaliation from their peers. They are also in touch with society itself, through its social organs (*i.e.* social institutions). Thanks to

---

6   Émile Durkheim, *The Division of Labour in Society*, trans. by Wilfred D. Halls, ed.
     by Steven Lukes (Hampshire, Palgrave Macmillan, 2013, 2nd edn.), pp. 57–84.
7   *Ibid.*, pp. 88–103.

positive rights contained in restitutive law, the human individual takes on increased importance within organic solidarity. Mechanical solidarity still survives within modern society, as one can observe in the subsistence of ethnic, religious, friendly communities, and the like.

On a preliminary basis it is worth mentioning that for Durkheim the rise of individualism is not due to any specific historical conjuncture.

> Individualism and free thinking are of no recent date, neither from 1789, the Reformation, scholasticism, the collapse of Graeco-Latin polytheism, nor the fall of oriental theocracies. They are a phenomenon that has no fixed starting point but one that has developed unceasingly throughout history.[8]

However, on the basis of Durkheim's work, sociologist Hans Joas (2013) has shown that, throughout Western history, the progressive sacralisation of the human person has complemented a cultural shift, especially salient during the eighteenth century, which gave birth to human rights and reformed the penal system by opposing slavery and torture. Quoting Durkheim,[9] Joas suggests that human rights and human dignity should be regarded as the "religion of modernity".[10] Other celebrated thinkers have previously sketched important theories of modern identity — such as Georg Simmel,[11] Michel Foucault,[12] and Charles Taylor[13]. But Joas' account of the modern person, also taken in by sociologist Randall Collins (1992), is especially relevant here as it stems from Durkheim's theory of social rituals.

---

8   Durkheim, *The Division of Labour in Society*, p. 133.
9   Émile Durkheim, 'Individualism and the Intellectuals', In *Durkheim on Religion*, ed. by William S. F. Pickering (London: Routledge, 1975) 59–73 (pp. 61–62): "The human person, whose definition serves as the touchstone according to which good must be distinguished from evil, is considered as sacred, in what one might call the ritual sense of the word. It has something of that transcendent majesty which the churches of all times have given to their Gods. [...] Whoever makes an attempt on a man's life, on a man's liberty, on a man's honour inspires us with a feeling of horror, in every way analogous to that which the believer experiences when he sees his idol profaned". (amended translation)
10   Hans Joas, *The Sacredness of the Person. A New Genealogy of Human Rights*, trans. by Alex Skinner (Washington, DC: Georgetown University Press, 2013), pp. 49–50.
11   Georg Simmel, *On Individuality and Social Forms*, ed. by Donald N. Levine (Chicago: The University of Chicago Press, 1971).
12   Michel Foucault, *Surveiller et punir, Naissance de la prison* (Paris: Gallimard, 1975).
13   Charles Taylor, *Sources of the Self, The Making of the Modern Identity* (Cambridge, MA: Harvard University Press, 1989; repr. 2001).

Through a process of integration where more and more people are recognized as having a self (*i.e.* rationality, soul, etc.), it becomes an increasingly universal and sacred value. Yet the sacralisation of the person does not annihilate altogether penal measures and sanctions when it comes to criminal behaviour. In fact, violent punishments and disciplinarian techniques remain valid rituals designed to raise awareness about social values. They revive the collective respect for common beliefs and thereby reinforce society's identity, which manifests through collective sentiments. For that matter, even slavery is nowadays justified in an underhanded manner, coated in socially acceptable values ranging from correction and education to vocation and heroism: modern slavery is being called by other names like 'prison labour', 'bond labour', 'child labour', and other types of wage work also come close to slavery, such as domestic work and, since the beginning of the pandemic, essential work.

The sacralisation of the person gives rise to the modern identity of human beings, as most people know it today. Our moral compass generally reflects this sacralisation, as Taylor points out: The 'respect of life, integrity, and well-being' of others have become a set of non-negotiable moral standards, expected from all members of modern societies; these demands "are the ones we infringe when we kill or maim others, steal their property, strike fear into them and rob them of peace, or even refrain from helping them when they are in distress."[14] However, interestingly enough, our modern identity is actually taking place both *thanks to* and *in spite of* society, as Collins illustrates in a passage where he agrees with Goffman:

> We continually emphasize that we are giving our own opinions, not acting out some external role. Joking and irony are very popular ways of speaking today; these are ways of demonstrating that we can maintain a psychological detachment from the pressures and social organizations around us. Complaining and criticizing, [which are] other very popular conversational activities, are yet more ways of keeping ourselves independent. [...] All this constitutes a kind of cult of the ultra-self, demonstrating that you can produce endless layers of inner detachment from everything that other people can throw at you.[15]

The ambiguous relationship between individual and society is not easily explainable on the grounds of Durkheim's social theory. According to it, cynicism towards dominant social values, on which penal law and

---

14   *Ibid.*, p. 4.
15   Randall Collins, *Sociological insight; An Introduction to Non-Obvious Sociology* (New York: Oxford University Press, 1992, 2nd edn.), pp. 55–56.

social organs are based, is seen as a symptom of pathological perversion.[16] Collins already criticized Durkheim's 'functionalist' view of society as an organism, where each social institution would contribute to social order: He argues instead for an approach inspired by Weber and Marx, stressing the role of 'conflict and domination' among social groups and classes.[17] It is not rare indeed to observe that social organs do not always cooperate and that they occasionally even enter in conflict, often at the expense of the particular individuals who resorted to them in the first place. Nevertheless people have to rely on society for the protection of their rights, which is why they need to fit in and act in solidarity so as to gain credit and legitimacy. At the same time, personal accountability in front of the law puts the focus on individual actions, and this drives people to be competitive in the defence of their rights and the upliftment of their social status. So while solidarity bolsters collective sentiments, competitiveness regulates self-esteem.[18]

2. Habit in modern sacralisation rituals

The ambivalent relationship between individual and society requires adjustments, one of them being the creation of personality. Referring to the etymology of the word *person*, Goffman quotes Park on the analogy between the social self and a theatre mask, highlighting the idea that one *becomes* a person, as opposed to *being born* such.

> It is probably no mere historical accident that the word person, in its first meaning, is a mask [...] In a sense, and in so far as this mask represents the conception we have formed of ourselves — the role we are striving to live up to — this mask is our truer self, the self we would like to be. In the end, our conception of our role becomes second nature and an integral part of our personality. We come into the world as individuals, achieve character, and become persons.[19]

---

16   Durkheim, *The Division of Labour in Society*, p. 60.
17   Collins, *Sociological Insight*, p. 7.
18   Competitiveness is central in Simmel's account of the rise of individualism as well. On the eighteenth century premises of equality and freedom, Western demographic growth and the consequential establishment of cash economy separated the individual from the group, creating competitiveness and differentiation. See: Simmel, *On Individuality and Social Forms*, pp. 225, 277.
19   Robert Ezra Park, *Race and Culture* (Glencoe: The Free Press, 1950), pp. 249–50.

According to Goffman, one of the most important rituals that people have been performing in modern day is therefore that of engaging in the social game of expression and impression.[20] Expressing oneself is indeed a constitutive element of our present-day societies, because the self has become an object of worship. Goffman subscribes to Durkheim's view, quoting him as follows: 'the human personality is a sacred thing; one does not violate it nor infringe its bounds, while at the same time the greatest good is in communion with others'.[21] But Goffman then formulates things in a bolder way, saying that there is indeed no other *reality* to the self, than the social self.

> [W]hen the individual presents himself before others, his performance will tend to incorporate and exemplify the officially accredited values of the society, more so, in fact than does his behaviour as a whole. [...] To stay in one's room away from the place where the party is given, or away from where the practitioner attends to his client, is to stay away from where the reality is being performed. The world, in truth, is a wedding.[22]

In this mind-set it is not sufficient for an individual to *have* freedom and opinions: one must *exhibit* them too. Social life before pandemic occurred was characterised by a set of habitual practices that would meet people's needs when it comes to affirming their personality by demonstrating autonomy and integrity. Most people would have the opportunity to socialize daily. Groups used to gather in various kinds of activities, displaying what Durkheim calls "rituals".[23] Working in team, having lunch with colleagues, going shopping with friends, meeting new people at a party, or dating; any of the above would potentially satisfy an individual's need for peer recognition and self-esteem regulation, while simultaneously enhance work and consumption behaviour. Therefore engaging in community life would not necessarily interfere with the broader social system, quite the contrary.

Like Durkheim, Goffman conceives the performances that highlight the common values of society as ceremonies. They reaffirm and revive the existence of the community while also paying tribute to the individual as a sacred thing. There are several states of ritual in the secular life: it can be

---

20 Erving Goffman, *The Presentation of Self in Everyday Life* (Edinburgh: University of Edinburgh, 1956), p. 2.
21 Durkheim, *Sociology and Philosophy*, tr. by D. F. Pocock, (Abingdon: Routledge, 2010), p. 17.
22 Goffman, *The Presentation of Self in Everyday Life*, p. 23.
23 Durkheim, *The Elementary Forms of Religious Life*.

"formal social activity, work, informal recreation, celebrating a new phase in the season cycle or in the life-cycle".[24] Goffman also talks about sexual intercourse as "part of the ceremonial system, a reciprocal ritual performed to confirm symbolically an exclusive social relationship".[25] So, reality is redefined and reassessed each time common values are being celebrated. Isolation from these ceremonies equals missing out on reality — the same reality, through which the self is being celebrated.

Of course, sophisticated manners, social distancing, and even absence are considered to be performances as well, typically for people who wish to distinguish themselves from others by avoiding familiar contact, creating even more difference or a downright aura of mystery.[26] Among the social roles available, Goffman identifies the performers (social actors belonging to a group), the audience (group members watching performers' interaction), the outsiders (audience or performers that are not group members), and the 'non-person'. The "classic type of non-person in our society is the servant", Goffman writes, but non-persons are also "the very young, the very old, the sick" as well as all the people "who play a technical role during important ceremonies but who are not, in a sense, treated as if present".[27] Interestingly enough, 'non-persons' are not necessarily unimportant. There are absent people who can obtain, through non-persons, all the information about social interactions, unbeknownst to performers or audience.[28]

In Goffman's terms, a person is a performer who builds their role in response to the social context that puts them on stage. Between sincerity and cynicism, the individual exists through the particular roles they perform, and thereby contributes to defining various social realities in which they are being involved. On their part, the audience and bystanders evaluate the performance based on many parameters. During face-to-face interaction, a lot of this distinction happens through unofficial communication, which

> may be carried on by innuendo, mimicked accents, well-placed jokes, significant pauses, veiled hints, purposeful kidding, expressive overtones, and many other sign practices. Rules regarding this laxity are quite strict.[29]

---

24 Goffman, *The Presentation of Self in Everyday Life*, p. 15.
25 *Ibid.*, p. 123, n. 1.
26 *Ibid.*, pp. 44–45.
27 *Ibid.*, pp. 95–96.
28 "It would seem that the role of non-person usually carries with it some subordination and disrespect, but we must not underestimate the degree to which the person who is given or who takes such a role can use it as a defence". *Ibid.*, p. 96.
29 *Ibid.*, p. 121.

In addition to the relatively close sphere in which verbal and non-verbal languages are staged, the main feature of rituals is, of course, their habitual nature. Most of daily life rituals are not consciously executed as ceremonies, but their disruption can be experienced as a scandal, because their habitual nature is bound to our sense of self. Collins, who endorses Goffman's view on the dramaturgical expression of the self, points out that repetition is key in the worship of shared values, as it is only this way that individuals can recharge their emotional batteries and group vitality is maintained.

> [T]he feeling of exaltation and emotional strength that comes from the group could not survive if the group did not reassemble before too much time elapses. The emotion-producing machine has to be run intermittently since its charges run down in between times.[30]

This being said, the model of the self as a performer amounts to a 'bureaucratization of the spirit' that typically hinders the expression of people's genuine, fluctuating moods. It contributes to the 'contemporary malaise', in which people lose their spontaneity as the social world, paradoxically, loses its reality.[31] Initially, social media may thus appear as an escape from social shallowness, because Internet users can create anonymous accounts to share intimate content. But social media platforms are designed in such a way that they can alter users' self-concepts[32] and self-esteem.[33] So, there are rituals for all stages and back-stages, and whether it is online or offline, individuals change role according to the situation.

Given such an interpretative framework, common people (as opposed to public figures) may be seen as assuming the role of audience or non-person with respect to public affairs, and even more so during the pandemic. Relatedly the virus outbreak may be seen as a counter-value against which social organs are carrying out public performances consisting in restricting individuals' freedom. At the same time, individuals are wrestling with the new constraints representing a counter-value to their own modern identity.

---

30   Collins, *Sociological Insight*, p. 43.
31   Christopher Lash, *The Culture of Narcissism. American Life in an Age of Diminishing Expectations* (New York: Norton, 1979), pp. 90–91.
32   Alexa K. Fox and others, 'Selfie-marketing: exploring narcissism and self-concept in visual user-generated content on social media', *Journal of Consumer Marketing*, 35(1) (2018), 11–21.
33   Hawi S. Nazir and Maya Samaha, 'The Relations Among Social Media Addiction, Self-Esteem, and Life Satisfaction in University Students', *Social Science Computer Review*, 35(5) (2017), 576–86.

3. *Modern sacred rituals versus 'healthy' pandemic habits*

In modern society, where rituals of sacralisation consist in social interactions, the reality of the self fluctuates as interactions may be spaced apart in time. Unlike in a community, whose homogeneity and fixed identity generates stability in the members' self-conception, the division of labour characterizing modern society implies a need to distinguish oneself. The tendency to specialize in a certain career or field of expertise comes with the need of being recognized as competent in such field. Therefore, despite the increase in autonomy deriving from the rise of individualism, the modern self is more than ever dependent on the recognition and validation of third parties, when it comes to its self-conception (identity) and self-esteem (sacredness). And the marketplace where social validation bits are being exchanged is none other than social interactions.

In line with Goffman's interpretation of social interactions both as a type of dramaturgical performance and as a ceremony, details are taking on great importance. While dialogues and behaviour are fundamental, facial expressions and voice tone also play a great part. In fact, they may represent the most important part, as they determine whether an individual can be trusted as a performer in the social game — at least for a while.

> When an individual passes such a test of expression-control, whether he receives it from his new team-mates in a spirit of jest, or from an unexpected necessity of playing in a serious performance, he can thereafter venture forth as a player who can trust himself and be trusted by others.[34]

The virus outbreak is obviously disrupting the codes of all these self-related modern rituals. So on top of the infection and death rates, the poor hospital conditions that many patients must endure, and the global economic desperation resulting from the attempts to contain the pandemic, the virus deeply affects everybody as a person. Waiting for successful vaccination to be carried out, the response to the outbreak has been to introduce hygiene practices ranging from personal sphere to interpersonal relations. If we consider also the limited access to public spaces and the restrictions concerning border crossing and curfews, our habits have been unsettled on many fronts. The situation is puzzling, as these healthy habits feel wrong and disrespectful to people's favourite ritual that sacralise their individual autonomy. Here are a few examples.

---

34   Goffman, *The Presentation of Self in Everyday Life*, p. 138.

Mandatory facemasks hide facial features and expressions, making it difficult to recognize one another. When it is not with the mask people are meeting online, but they can no longer rely on old codes of interaction, because they don't necessarily see their interlocutors; it is not clear whom they are talking to; and they don't know for sure whether the audience is listening. Also, the requirement to only run essential errands prevents people from going shopping as much as they used to. They can no longer fully exert their purchase power, which is a marker of their status.[35] A further example is social distancing and remote working, which enable less direct affirmation and recognition with respect to friends and co-workers. On the flip side, it is no longer possible for people to distinguish themselves by being socially distant on purpose, because everybody is socially distant. Finally, isolation or lockdown at home is quite simply unbearable for a lot of people, partly because significant rituals — such as morning routines — only make sense in the prospect of going out of the house.

The new form of social control represented by mandatory curfews, lockdowns and unemployment leaves little room for expressing oneself the old-fashioned way. Since people are relying on communication technologies so as to work from home — for those who still work —, they can reasonably be expected to be more present on social media. In an attempt to compensate for social distancing (and also because social media have become a new normal way of communicating), people try to revive their social self by engaging in online interactions, expressing opinions, sharing visual content, news or conspiracy theories.

It is when habits are disrupted that consciousness awakes, as Durkheim writes, through feelings of "uncertainty, tension, and anxiety".[36] The safety

---

35 Durkheim did not overlook the question of fashion, clothes, beard cut, and so on. (Durkheim, *The Division of Labour in Society*, p. 262) Simmel also considered fashion as a way to distinguish oneself, by introducing a trend, following it, or ignoring it altogether. (Simmel, *On Individuality and Social Forms*, pp. 294–323) Goffman follows them both, saying that "the most important piece of sign equipment associated with social class consists of the status symbols through which material wealth is expressed." (Goffman, *The Presentation of Self in Everyday Life*, p. 24).

36 "Let us imagine an organism which finds everything it needs in the milieu in which it lives. It will function mechanically. Consciousness will not appear, as there will be no need for it. [...] | As soon as there is tension or conflict, however, the situation changes. If the animal does not find what it needs, [...] it has to seek the new something which contains what it needs, it has to 'reflect', to wonder where it will find it. [...] Reflective thought, or 'knowledge', appears in very special conditions, at a cross-roads situation in which the being is faced with a whole range of possible solutions. And in such situation, what are our feelings?

paradox arises from the fact that virus prevention focuses on physical health to the expense of psychosocial needs, thereby doing violence to habits that were deeply engrained in communities as well as in our modern identity. This paradox is a breach within social solidarity, where social bounds are jeopardized in order to maintain the smooth functioning of healthcare facilities. In Durkheimian terms we can interpret this phenomenon as a tension between mechanical and organic solidarity: community life is interrupted, so that the health care system is less overwhelmed.

The case of undermined religious cults is iconic, but the safety paradox is salient in many secular cases too, such as the accompaniment of the sick and the dying. Because of the contagiousness of the virus, infected patients are being isolated from their own families, kids separated from their parents, grandparents from their children and grandchildren — some of them ending up passing away alone, without ever seeing a friendly or familiar face again. Even the fundamental social ritual of mourning is subject to restrictive policies imposing the observance of rules, such as keeping empty spaces between mourners, and limiting their number at the funeral. These additional rules do not contribute to the ritual itself. They are meant to inhibit the virus spread, but in fact they also hinder a ritual that Durkheim sees as crucial for increasing social vitality.

> The basis of mourning is the impression of enfeeblement that is felt by the group when it loses a member. But this very impression has the effect of bringing the individuals close to one another, putting them into closer touch, and inducing in them the same state of soul. And from all this comes a sensation of renewed strength, which counteracts the original enfeeblement. People cry together because they continue to be precious to one another and because, regardless of the blow that has fallen upon it, the collectivity is not breached.[37]

Present-day rituals of sacralisation are of course not limited to what is referred to by Durkheim or Goffman in their own day. The pandemic itself offers new opportunities of carrying out rituals of solidarity, in which individuals can also affirm their integrity and autonomy. Such are/were the habit of applauding the medical staff at the window on evenings, wearing customized or matching masks, meeting online for seminars, to play games, or drink. New habits may also include going out beyond curfew time, secretly gathering in bigger groups than allowed, and so on.

Uncertainty, tension, anxiety". Durkheim, *Pragmatism and Sociology*, trans. by J. C. Whitehouse (Cambridge: Cambridge University Press, 1983), pp. 37–38.

37   Durkheim, *The Elementary Forms of Religious Life*, p. 405.

Conclusion

Disruption of social interactions has a negative impact on self-conception, because personality is deeply involved in the identification with a social role; therefore pandemic habits, by disrupting face-to-face interactions, affect individual personality.[38] We may ask ourselves indeed whether collectivity is breached under these circumstances. At the same time, travel restrictions and news about the way countries are dealing with vaccination raise collective feelings pertaining to people's national identities. It is thus possible to talk in terms of social solidarity, at a national level, in the war against the virus.[39] In so far as this global public health challenge requires selflessness, most people are compelled to assume the role of 'non-persons' in public, and then feel the need to compensate through other avenues, including social media. This ability to assume different subsequent roles can be explained by the fluidity of self-concept.[40] However, although recent research suggests that social media open a space for rituals between group members, these rituals cannot altogether replace face-to-face interactions, in particular because this type of long-distance communication generates misunderstandings.[41]

The Durkheimian theory of social rituals can be invoked, as Goffman does, to describe codified face-to-face interactions pertaining to community life and modern society. These models are associated to solidarity, mechanical and organic. But against the background of present-day pandemic restrictions, the same cannot be said about rituals on social media. The existence of these platforms is motivated by business interests, which are not concerned about the human need for contact and intimacy. The way they are designed actually fosters isolation because the users separate

---

38   Goffman, *The Presentation of Self in Everyday Life*, p. 156.
39   Christopher M. Federico, Agnieszka Golec de Zavala, and Tomasz Baran, 'Collective Narcissism, In-Group Satisfaction, and Solidarity in the Face of COVID-19', *Social Psychological and Personality Science*, 12(6), (2021), 1071–1081 (first published: October 14th, 2020).
40   Rina S. Onorato and John C. Turner, 'Fluidity in the self-concept: the shift from personal to social identity', *European Journal of Social Psychology*, 34 (2004), 257–78.
41   Susan Abel, Tanya Macin, and Charlotte Brownlow, 'Social media, rituals, and long-distance family relationship maintenance: A mixed-methods systematic review', *New Media & Society*, 23(3), (2021), 632–54 (first published: September 14th, 2020); Ayla G. Lopez and Kennet G. Cuarteros, 'Exploring the Effects of Social Media on Interpersonal Communication among Family Members', *Canadian Journal of Family and Youth*, 12(1), (2020), 60–80.

themselves from direct environment, and competitiveness is encouraged by way of upvote scores.[42] The power of these contrivances is to create ostracism under the guise of integration, by establishing a gap between people who use social media and those who don't. Furthermore they are designed to generate user habits, such as that of remaining connected.

> Anything that obliges our activity to take on a definite form can give rise to habits that result in dispositions which then have to be satisfied. Moreover, these dispositions alone are truly fundamental.[43]

While teleworking and video calls represent a substitute for real life encounters, people also become more exposed to using social media, the habitual use of which covertly reinforces isolation. As long as people need communities and social environment made of carbon-based life in order to ensure the sacredness of their self, the habits of social distancing and social media cannot be considered sustainable. It seems fair to expect that the massive use, under pandemic restrictions, of communication technologies including social media will have consequences reaching beyond the end of the pandemic.

Yet the advantages of teleworking should not be dismissed, as it saves people commuting time and enables them to attend online events taking place in locations that would be burdensome to physically reach. Relatedly, recorded lectures and conferences allow for a wider and more effective diffusion of knowledge, as real-life events may be full of distractions. Finally, it is conceivable that the interface of communication technologies may actually be more convenient to people who don't feel easily sociable.

The 'uncertainty, tension', and 'anxiety' ascribed by Durkheim to the state in which conscience and reflective thinking arise, in the circumstances of pandemic restrictions and the impossibility to indulge as much in sacralising rituals, shows the vulnerability of the social self. But as much as the social self may appear shallow and prone to collapse without the support of social interactions, a deeper self can be seen underneath, ready to take up the challenge of the change in habits and come up with innovative solutions.

---

42   More than isolation, research actually shows correlation between the use social media and depression. Anthony Robinson and others, 'Social comparisons, social media addiction, and social interaction: An examination of specific social media behaviors related to major depressive disorder in a millennial population', *Journal of Applied Biobehavioral Research*, 24(1), (2019), 1–14.

43   Durkheim, *The Division of Labour in Society*, p. 65.

DENISE VINCENTI

EPIDEMIC PSYCHOSIS
Suggestion and Psychological Contagion in the Reflections of Giuseppe Sergi (1841–1936)

1. *Introduction*

Analyzing the sociological, political, and psychological impact of the COVID-19 pandemic through the concepts of fear and disruption seems not only crucial for the understanding of the current situation, but also philosophically fruitful, as it entails a reflection on the way in which human interactions and external factors shape an individual's sphere. As far as extraordinary and upsetting events are concerned, what appears to be of greatest interest is precisely the nexus between individuality and collectivity, between an individual's identity (psychologically, emotionally, and morally speaking) and the identity of the group to which they belong. An interesting case study is represented by the change of consolidated and habitual behaviors. If it is true, as William James remarks, that habit is not a second nature but 'ten times nature',[1] meaning that it is harder to break a habit than to acquire a new one, it is even more startling that some events manage to produce sudden and enduring changes in our lives and routines. From a philosophical and psychological standpoint, that is a crucial question, since such changes seem to stem from some powerful and hidden motivations, such as the influence of the group on the individual. To what extent do fearful and unexpected events, like the outbreak of the COVID-19 pandemic, enable the emergence of collective behaviors and beliefs, which tend to erase individual identity? Does fear facilitate the creation of shared patterns of conduct, which we unknowingly conform to?

There is a natural tendency in human beings to conform to certain collective behaviors, in particular when strong feelings (fear, panic, bewilderment) tend to put a strain on our judgment. People experienced such a psychological phenomenon especially during the first months of the pandemic, when media, newspapers, physicians or politicians

---

1   William James, *The Principles of Psychology*, 2 vols (London: MacMillan, 1890), 1, p. 136.

recommended to adopt precautionary actions — often in striking opposition to their ordinary habits — in order to reduce the risk of contagion. Even if the information provided was not always consistent or clear, people listened to these suggestions and changed their behaviors in accordance with them. One could easily explain it by resorting to the sense of trust people had toward the scientific community or their political leaders. But, alongside the rather widespread acceptance of new rules and conducts of life, we have also witnessed the emergence of some rather concerning mass phenomena, such as the spreading of negationist movements and conspiracy theories. These phenomena appear to be different in nature from the former ones. They derive, indeed, from a deep sense of distrust toward the institutional channels of communication, and they claim to be free from any external conditioning or influence. Yet, it is possible to suppose a common psychological source for both phenomena. As scholars of collective psychology have argued since the field's rise in the last decades of the nineteenth century, the influence of the group on the individual can be regarded as a pivotal factor in the emergence of new patterns of behavior and the disruption of consolidated habits. In this paper, I will attempt to further this hypothesis, by resorting to a conceptualization of the late nineteenth century Italian psychologist Giuseppe Sergi's notion of 'epidemic psychosis' (*psicosi epidemica*). Such a conceptualization could provide fruitful insights on the psychological dynamics engendering and regulating phenomena such as the emergence of collective behaviors or the spread of commonly-held ideas, beliefs, fears, and concerns. Furthermore, the relationship established by Sergi between abnormal behaviors and the notion of 'epidemic' can enlighten the current situation, since it not only indicates a psychosis caused by the outbreak of an epidemic, but also a psychosis conceived per se as a spreading epidemic.

2. *Criminal crowd and degeneration: Taine, Lombroso and Sergi*

The idea that the crowd is not merely the sum of individual behaviors and thoughts but an actual entity, provided with its own beliefs, volitions and ideas, is usually ascribed to Gustave Le Bon's 1895 text *La psychologie des foules*,[2] considered to be a groundbreaking study on social and collective psychology. Such a conception represents nevertheless a rather widespread topic within the nineteenth century scientific community, especially with

---

2   Gustave Le Bon, *La psychologie des foules* (Paris: Alcan, 1895).

regard to its psychological and anthropological implications.[3] Some anticipations of this idea can be found, for instance, in Hippolyte Taine's *Les origines de la France contemporaine*,[4] where the analysis of the eighteenth- and nineteenth century French revolutionary movements is based on a psychological study of the crowd's role in the outbreak of the revolutions — with a focus on the criminals' influence on such historical events. Likewise, Gabriel Tarde's mimetic anthropology, postulating the law of imitation as the fundamental phenomenon which constitutes social life, represents another pivotal theorization fostering the rise of the study on collective behaviors.[5]

Generally speaking, the idea that an individual's identity tends to dissolve into that of the group, gradually losing its peculiarity and singularity, seems to have exerted a powerful fascination on several psychologists, anthropologists, and sociologists of the time, arguably as a response to the need to understand the changes which their political and social environments were undergoing. It is no surprise indeed that in Taine's enquiry, aimed at detecting the historical, sociological, and psychological factors leading to the French defeat in the Franco–Prussian war, by analyzing the history of France's political instability and the role played by crowds in these events, the Parisian facts of September 4th, 1870 stood as a testament to the people's influence on major political changes. In particular, Taine conceived of France's recent past as the result of a broader social and psychical degeneration: his historical account drew attention to the pivotal role of criminal leaders (e.g., Jacobins) and crowds — depicted

---

3   See, e.g., Olivier Bosc, *La foule criminelle: positivisme, politique et criminologie en Italie et en France à la fin du XIXe siècle. Scipio Sighele (1868-1913) et l'école lombrosienne* (Paris IX-Dauphine: Thèse de doctorat en science politique, 2001); Olivier Bosc, 'De la *folla delinquente* à la *follacultura*: Scipio Sighele e Pasquale Rossi prophètes italiens de la modernité au tournant du siècle', *Laboratoire italien — Politique et société*, 4 (2003), pp. 37–56; Damiano Palano, *Il potere della moltitudine: l'invenzione dell'inconscio collettivo nella teoria politica e nelle scienze sociali italiane tra Otto e Novecento* (Milan: Vita e Pensiero, 2002); Emilia Musumeci, *Emozioni, crimine, giustizia: un'indagine storico-giuridica tra Otto e Novecento* (Milan: FrancoAngeli, 2015); Michela Nacci, 'La psychologie collective', *Revue historique*, 1 (2016), pp. 129–38.
4   Hippolyte Taine, *Les origines de la France contemporaine*, 5 vols (Paris: Hachette, 1875–1893).
5   Gabriel Tarde, *Les lois de l'imitation: étude sociologique* (Paris: Alcan, 1890). As far as this inaugural phase of collective psychology is concerned, we should also mention Prosper Despine (*moral contagion*), Alfred Espinas (*collective suggestion*), Enrico Ferri (*psychological fermentation*), Scipio Sighele (*criminal crowd*), and other thinkers.

130   *Disruption of Habits during the Pandemic*

as bloodthirsty and heinous hordes — in the events that occurred between 1789 and 1870.[6]

The analysis of the criminal crowd as a powerful political and sociological agent also lies at the center of Italian criminal anthropologist Cesare Lombroso's work. In a text written in 1890 with Rodolfo Laschi,[7] Lombroso postulated that political insurrections were achieved by some exceptional and deranged men (*degenerati*), who managed to influence and lead large numbers of people. Relying on his theory of crime's genesis formulated in *L'uomo delinquente*,[8] Lombroso stated that political events had their roots in biological factors (as the phenomenon of *degeneration*), triggered by social, climatic, racial, sexual, economic, political, and individual dynamics. As for Taine, along with Lombroso, the diagnostic category of 'degeneration', introduced by the French psychiatrist Bénédict Augustin Morel,[9] represented a keystone in the explanation of collective behaviors and socio-political changes. Although the term 'degeneration' was initially employed to explain the increase of sickness, mental disorders, and criminal tendencies in patients with mental retardation, it became a much broader category, relevant for non-psychiatric subjects. Morel's idea that psychological and behavioral impairments were caused by inheritable physical abnormalities that worsened from generation to generation could not fail to attract thinkers like Taine and Lombroso, who embraced a reductionist approach in psychological and sociological matters, and stressed the importance of environmental factors and heredity in such questions.

In the same period, the Italian anthropologist and psychologist Giuseppe Sergi[10] emphasized, in turn, the role of degeneration in socio-political

6   See Palano, pp. 5, 28, 40, 147–49.
7   Cesare Lombroso and Rodolfo Laschi, *Il delitto politico e le rivoluzioni* (Turin: Fratelli Bocca, 1890).
8   Cesare Lombroso, *L'uomo delinquente in rapporto all'antropologia, alla medicina legale ed alle discipline carcerarie* (Turin: Fratelli Bocca, 1876).
9   Bénédict Augustin Morel, *Traité des dégénérescences physiques, intellectuelles et morales de l'espèce humaine* (Paris: Baillière, 1857); see also, Michel Coddens, 'La théorie de l'hérédité-dégénérescence: Morel, Lombroso, Magnan, et les autres', *L'An-Je Lacanien*, 2 (2016), pp. 129–49.
10 On the life and work of Giuseppe Sergi, see, e.g., Giuseppe Mucciarelli (ed.), *Giuseppe Sergi nella storia della psicologia e dell'antropologia in Italia* (Bologna: Pitagora, 1987); Vincenzo Bongiorno, 'Giuseppe Sergi', in Guido Cimino and Nino Dazzi (eds.), *La psicologia in Italia* (Milan: LED, 1998), pp. 109–57; Elisabetta Cicciola, 'The Origins of Psychology in Rome: the Contribution of Giuseppe Sergi', in Jaap Bos and Maria Sinatra (eds.), *The History of the Human Sciences: An Open Atmosphere* (Lecce: Pensa Multimedia, 2010), pp. 92–101;

dynamics. As Sergi would openly acknowledge in 1906,[11] his research in the 1880s on degeneration were inspired by Lombroso's theory, especially with regard to the nexus between degeneration and criminality. Sergi resorts to these ideas already in 1883, in a study on 'the stratification of character' (*stratificazione del carattere*),[12] and afterwards in 1885 in his text *L'origine dei fenomeni psichici*,[13] but it is only in 1889 that he decides to devote an entire work to the topic. In *Le degenerazioni umane*, Sergi indeed identifies three causes of degeneration: 1. regression as a result of prehuman or beastly atavism; 2. morbid congenital conditions (inherited) or accidental factors occurred during conception or intrauterine life; and 3. external conditions which affect an individual's physical and mental development.[14] All these causes are biological, meaning that they depend on physical or organic impairments. Even the third kind of degeneration, albeit caused by external conditions (e.g., social factors, poor education, poverty, alcoholism, etc.), cannot be considered as totally independent from the individual's physical constitution. Although these forms of degenerations do not affect all human beings (for instance, atavism is typical of those affected by microcephalia),[15] according to Sergi an individual's character is the result of multiple stratifications, which include not only the features acquired through experience, education and social interactions, but also all sorts of atavistic, pre-human, and inherited pathological traits.[16] This allows him to explain why, in certain circumstances, like in the frenzy of the crowd or during insurrections, even the most cultivated person could

Luca Tedesco, *Giuseppe Sergi e la morale fondata sulla scienza: degenerazione e perfezionamento razziale* (Milan: Unicopli, 2012); Alessandro Volpone, 'Giuseppe Sergi "Champion" of Darwinism', *Journal of Anthropological Sciences*, 89 (2011), pp. 59–69; Giovanni Cerro, 'Giuseppe Sergi. 'The Portrait of a Positivist Scientist', *Journal of Anthropological Sciences*, 95 (2017), pp. 109–36.

11 Giuseppe Sergi, 'I caratteri degenerativi nell'uomo secondo Cesare Lombroso', in Giuseppe Amadei and others (ed.), *L'opera di Cesare Lombroso nella scienza e nelle sue applicazioni*, 2nd edn (Milan-Turin-Rome: Fratelli Bocca, 1908), p. 36. See also, Tedesco, pp. 41–46.

12 Giuseppe Sergi, *La stratificazione del carattere e la delinquenza* (Milan: Dumolard, 1883).

13 Giuseppe Sergi, *L'origine dei fenomeni psichici e la loro significazione biologica* (Milan: Dumolard, 1885).

14 Giuseppe Sergi, *Le degenerazioni umane* (Milan: Dumolard, 1889), p. 26. On Sergi's studies on degeneration, see, e.g., Lino Rossi, 'Il problema delle degenerazioni umane nell'antropologia psicologica di Giuseppe Sergi', in Mucciarelli (ed.), pp. 63–81; Tedesco, pp. 41–54.

15 Sergi, *Le degenerazioni umane*, p. 28.

16 *Ibid.*, pp. 35–8.

act brutally. This phenomenon can be described as a recrudescence of atavist instincts.[17]

Yet, alongside Sergi's monistic and reductionist perspective, what has to be highlighted in this theory is the idea that such degenerations, in addition to producing terrible effects on vital functions, also generate intellectual and moral degenerations which affect society itself.[18] There is, indeed, a sort of isomorphism between societies and their members, to the point that the evolution (or degeneration) of individuals deeply impacts social evolution (or degeneration):

> There is an evolution in human societies, and this evolution starts from the people who constitute societies. After a certain amount of time, societies undergo a change, and that change is accomplished *pari passu* with that of society in some individuals, it is delayed in others, and achieved in advance by pioneers.[19]

Societies and individuals are, in Sergi's view, conceivable as living organisms: they form, develop, die, and most importantly, vary in relation to external or internal influences.[20] Between them, a sort of osmotic relationship ensures that a change in the individuals' constitution produces a correspondent effect in the structure of society, and vice versa. That amounts to say that a society is not merely the sum of its members. Rather, there is a profound correspondence between the two, as the correspondence joining the body to its constitutive parts. If a disease affects one organ, the entire body is affected; likewise, a general state of health is required so that every single organ could exercise its own function.

As in the case of bodily parts, the members of a society can be described as constitutive elements of a whole, whose individuality constantly dissolves into the identity of the group. Without denying the specificity of each individual (their character, beliefs, ideas, etc.), Sergi aims to show how much the outlines of individuality are blurry and undefined. Individuals are centers of forces, not isolated substances, since the nature of the human psyche consists in being "easily inclined to the communicability of common actions, to solidarity, often with a certain annihilation of one's individual

---

17   *Ibid.*, pp. 85–118.
18   *Ibid.*, p. 26. See also, Cesare Rossi, 'Giuseppe Sergi e la psicologia sociale in Italia', in Mucciarelli (ed.), pp. 51–62.
19   Sergi, *Le degenerazioni umane*, p. 37.
20   *Ibid.*, p. 33.

nature [*impronta individuale*]".²¹ But what makes this interconnection possible? What is responsible for this 'osmosis' between an individual and the group they belong to? Contrary to Lombroso's perspective, which mainly focused on the individual's loss of identity in criminal crowds and grounded this phenomenon in biological factors, Sergi not only decides to broaden the purview of his analysis to all social phenomena (both normal and pathological), but he also tries to offer a psychological account of the problem. What makes individuals constitutive parts of a whole and not isolated substances is that:

> The human psyche is subjected to that suggestive influence that we are used to exclusively attribute to a special, morbid phenomenon: hypnotism; actually, each phenomenon of our mental life is an example of suggestion [...]. A certain idea, announced by voice or in writing, is an actual suggestion; we absorb it and we let ourselves be carried away by it in our thoughts and actions [...]. Political, scientific, and religious proselytism are more or less complex effects of suggestion. The hypnotic state does not reveal a new condition of the psyche, but a deep disposition.²²

Suggestion, far from solely being a morbid phenomenon produced by hypnotism, is rather a general condition of the human psyche. And this deep disposition is what engenders the interconnection — in terms of thoughts, actions, beliefs, ideas, etc. — between the members of a society. The invisible bond that constitutes society as a whole is thus a psychological principle. As with the term 'degeneration', the notion of suggestion loses here its medical and psychiatric meaning, becoming a global phenomenon of the human mind. Upon closer inspection, Lombroso had already somehow pointed out the role of suggestion in collective behaviors, showing the effects of imitation and temporary madness on entire populations²³ — a study that drew upon Charcot's and Richer's accounts on the relationship between demonic possession and hysteria.²⁴ But the novelty of Sergi's reflection lies in the fact that suggestion is here provided with a universal value. In *Le degenerazioni umane*, this theorization is

21 *Ibid.*, p. 46.
22 *Ibid.*
23 Cesare Lombroso and Pietro Nocito, 'Davide Lazzaretti', *Archivio di psichiatria, antropologia criminale, e scienze penali*, 1 (1880), pp. 145–84; see also Palano, pp. 213–14.
24 Jean-Martin Charcot and Paul Richer, *Les démoniaques dans l'art* (Paris: Delahaye et Lecrosnier, 1887).

only sketched out: suggestion is indeed mentioned only to substantiate his idea of the permeability of human character, and to show the blurriness of the individual sphere. It becomes nevertheless fundamental in his later texts, where the main object of study is the influence of the group on the individual and the pathological outcomes of it.

3. *Epidemic psychosis*

One year before the publication of *Le degenerazioni umane*, Sergi had inaugurated his course at the Italian Institute of Anthropology in Rome with a lesson on a rather peculiar topic: the phenomenon of epidemic psychosis. This lesson will later become an article, featured in the 1889 issue of *Rivista di filosofia scientifica* — a pioneering Italian journal of scientific psychology and Positivist philosophy — and afterwards printed by the publishing house Dumolard as a separate book.[25] The significance of this study for Sergi is clear. In 1893, he decides to include this analysis in another book, *Per l'educazione del carattere*, where the problem of epidemic psychosis is addressed in relation to a more general enquiry on character formation and education.[26]

The point of departure is the same as in *Le degenerazioni umane*: human beings and societies have to be conceived as organisms, subjected to external and internal influences. From a methodological viewpoint, this means that true psychology should consist first and foremost in the study of collective thoughts and behaviors, instead of aimlessly focusing on individuals:

> Individual psychology has made much remarkable progress up to today, but it has a flaw: it studies humans as isolated beings, whereas, like each and every animal, they cannot be separated from the organic whole [...]. Human biology is like the biology of the organic kingdom; an individual's life is incomprehensible if not linked to the life of the animal group to which it belongs.[27]

---

25 Giuseppe Sergi, 'Psicosi epidemica', *Rivista di filosofia scientifica*, 8 (1889), pp. 151–73; then, *Psicosi epidemica* (Milan: Dumolard, 1889).
26 Giuseppe Sergi, *Per l'educazione del carattere*, 2nd edn (Milan: Dumolard, 1893), pp. 125–52.
27 *Ibid.*, pp. 125–26.

As an anthropologist and ethnologist, Sergi is fully aware that human beings are naturally inclined to gather in groups. In order to grasp what lies beneath social interaction, in the first part of his career Sergi had resorted to a set of conceptualizations issued from his anthropological studies, such as empathy, ethnical psyche, or the influence of stock (*stirpe*) on individuals.[28] Yet, in his study on epidemic psychosis, these notions are presented as negligible. They represent the manifestation of a more general and fundamental principle, which is not anthropological, but rather physio-psychological: the law of receptivity.[29]

The law of receptivity is, according to Sergi, universal, meaning that it does not exclusively pertain to human nature, but constitutes a general principle, regulating all aspects of reality, from physicochemical reactions to the most sophisticated processes of the mind. As William James remarks in a text on Sergi's psychology, such a conception has to be considered as an actual monistic approach to reality, where the transition from inorganic to organic matter, from vegetative to animal life, from perception to intellection is explained in terms of the 'transformation' of a unique and fundamental principle.[30] The same law that works beneath inorganic matter and biological phenomena also regulates the workings of the human mind. In Sergi's words, as every organic tissue enters into action because it is excited by an external stimulus, so the psyche has the ability to receive external impressions and display the provoked activity in the form of actions. *Receptivity* is precisely this ability to receive external impressions, whereas the ability to transform them into actions is called *reflection*.[31]

In this perspective, the human psyche is considered a center of forces, whose main activity consists of a rather mechanical work of transformation of impressions into actions. Although Sergi specifies that receptivity does not equate to passivity, since the reception of impressions is followed by a correspondent response,[32] it is clear that, in this theory, no spontaneous feeling, sensation, or perception is detectable in the human being.[33] Every psychical phenomenon is determined and conditioned by a certain stimulus (external or internal), which stands as the efficient cause of human

---

28   *Ibid.*, p. 126.
29   *Ibid.*, p. 127.
30   William James, '*Dolore e piacere: storia naturale dei sentimenti*. Giuseppe Sergi', *Psychological Review*, 2 (1895), pp. 601–04 (p. 602).
31   Sergi, *Per l'educazione del carattere*, p. 127.
32   *Ibid.*
33   *Ibid.*, p. 125.

sensations, movements, perceptions, ideas, thoughts, behaviors, and also beliefs.

Nevertheless, receptivity can display different levels of action. If considered in relation to the most basic phenomena of human life (sensations, perceptions, reflex movements), it is nothing more than a simple transformation of stimuli. It becomes much more articulated when it comes to complex psychological phenomena, which are determined not only by environmental factors, but also by social interactions. Living in a social group means to exposure to peer influence. And this influence deeply shapes an individual's identity, to the point that it is hard to draw a line of demarcation between what exclusively belongs to the individual and what results from their social environment. In order to qualify social influence, Sergi resorts to a conception that he had already employed in his previous works: *suggestion*. Suggestion and receptivity are not different laws or principles, since the former is a mere intensification of the latter.[34] Therefore, in lieu of being conceived as a special form of sympathy or empathy, suggestion should be regarded, like receptivity, as a mechanical law of the psyche. "The life of the psyche", Sergi states, "is really an actual automatism".[35] Human behaviors, thoughts, and beliefs are not spontaneous, but always provoked and induced. Likewise, human life can be compared to a constant state of hypnosis, except for the fact that the subject is awake and does not fall into a pathological dream state.[36] This condition, far from being exceptional, is a common trait of our everyday life:

> A thought expressed in a newspaper or an opinion formulated on current political facts are easily accepted by the readers, or at least by the majority of them; similarly, it is easy to find, in regard to a law which is under discussion, a certain consensus among favorable opinions and unfavorable ones. Let's consider the coming of a sovereign, the German emperor; newspapers start a campaign two months earlier to prepare his welcoming, and during these months they show off a series of ideas to have, emotions to feel, and needed courtesies to perform in honor of the ally, of the friend of the country, and promise feasts and enjoyments to the people. [...] The day of the sovereign's arrival, everybody is ready to welcome him and they seem to have spontaneously gathered without the need of any suggestion, although newspapers had competed to indicate the very moment of his arrival.[37]

---

34   *Ibid.*, pp. 128–29.
35   *Ibid.*, p. 129.
36   *Ibid.*, p. 130.
37   *Ibid.*

People gathering to celebrate the coming of the sovereign is not a spontaneous act, or the expression of personal preferences and convictions. Rather, it is the natural consequence of what we would call a 'mediatic campaign'. Nonetheless, suggestion does not produce complete homologation. As Sergi points out, responses to a same suggestion may vary according to individual predispositions. If it is true that some people, being keener to give in to external stimuli, immediately conform to a certain trend, others tend to resist. This depends on the degree of receptibility each individual has. Bodily constitution, hereditary traits, sex, and ethnicity, are just some of the factors that can influence a person's receptibility.[38] More than that, suggestion is not immediate. It can take some time before an idea can persuade an individual. Existing systems of thoughts, beliefs, and consolidated behaviors can reduce the effectiveness of external suggestions. Yet, according to Sergi, such an impediment is often temporary. Just as in the formation of new habits, repetition gradually replaces existing ideas and feelings with new ones. A sufficiently long exposure to a certain suggestion has the power to change even the most stubborn mind or resistant temper.[39]

Now, what can be said for an individual is also valid for groups, societies, or populations. Suggested ideas, emotions, and movements are able to spread and reach large numbers of people:

> This suggestion propagates as an epidemic, leaving some men utterly immune, some violently affected, others mildly. [...] I call it *epidemic psychosis*, precisely because the disease is psychological.[40]

Sergi's decision to employ the word 'psychosis' is quite interesting from a technical and classificatory viewpoint. Indeed, the term 'psychosis' indicates a severe mental disease, which profoundly alters the perception of reality, and hence requires thorough medical and psychiatric treatment. It is also worth noting that the end of the nineteenth century was characterized by the emergence of various classification systems of mental disorders. In Italy, the psychiatrist and anthropologist Enrico Morselli proposed in 1885 a new classification of mental diseases, focused on different kinds of psychoses (congenital, hereditary, acquired).[41] Interestingly enough, Morselli's system did not take into account the existence of collective

---

38 *Ibid.*, pp. 131–32.
39 *Ibid.*, pp. 132–33.
40 *Ibid.*, p. 137.
41 Enrico Morselli, *Manuale di semejotica delle malattie mentali*, 2 vols (Milan: Vallardi, 1885), 1, pp. 429–38. See also, Giuseppina Salomone and Raffaele

and general psychoses. It is thus fair to say that Sergi's study on epidemic psychosis not only shed light on a rather original and little-studied phenomenon, but also aimed to enrich existing classificatory systems with a new diagnostic category.

But what is precisely an epidemic psychosis? In Sergi's words, it is an 'epidemic of the human spirit'.[42] Like other devastating epidemics, such as plague or cholera, psychoses can spread and infect entire cities, nations or continents. A certain belief, expressed by a charismatic person or by a small group of highly persuasive people, can become the belief of the many. According to Sergi, such a spreading of ideas, emotions, and behaviors is an actual *contagion*, which nevertheless differs from the one occurring during 'regular' epidemics since it is solely psychological. This does not mean that its effects cannot be as severe or fatal as in regular epidemics. A deviant behavior, if shared by a large number of people, is a mortal threat to the well-being of individuals and societies.[43]

It is not clear if Sergi wants here to circumscribe the category of "epidemic psychosis" only to the spread of aberrant ideas and behaviors, or if he considers instead all psychological contagion to be negative. He distinctively states that every massive and uncontrolled spread of ideas should be regarded as an epidemic psychosis.[44] Thus, it seems that, for him, homologation is always to be avoided. On the other hand, the examples he provides only concern specific kinds of emotions, ideas, and behaviors. The outbreak of an epidemic psychosis is, indeed, fostered by some special conditions. Devastating epidemics, distressed economic and political conditions, frightening natural phenomena, religious feelings, and superstitions are just some of the events that, generating fear and discomfort, can lead the majority of people to act in a similar, deviant way. As Sergi recalls, during the Middle Ages, the outbreak of the black plague, increasing the mortality rate and the conditions of poverty, encouraged the formation of various cults, such as the cult of Flagellants (*Flagellanti*) in Italy, which attracted many people, seduced by their promise of redemption.[45]

This begs the question: *what are the triggering factors of an epidemic psychosis?* In general, we could say: all material and spiritual conditions able to cause distress and affliction. Exactly as in hypnotism, where

Arnone, 'La nosografia psichiatrica italiana prima di Kraepelin', *Giornale italiano di psicopatologia*, 15 (2009), pp. 75–88 (p. 85).

42   Sergi, *Per l'educazione del carattere*, p. 137.
43   *Ibid.*
44   *Ibid.*
45   *Ibid.*, p. 141.

suggestion only works if the subject's mind is ready to receive the hypnotic suggestion, so in epidemic psychoses some special conditions must be in place for the psychological contagion to take effect. Usually, physical and/ or mental vulnerability is sufficient to predispose individuals to suggestion. Such states are more frequent during exceptional events, where the uncertainty about the future ends up aggravating existing problems and distressed conditions.[46]

After having proven that psychological contagion requires a 'favorable' environment to produce effects on a global scale, Sergi decides to address the way in which epidemic psychosis works from a psychological standpoint:

> The first effect of the manifestation of strange and audacious ideas is a sort of *bewilderment* and *surprise*. Bewilderment is a curious psychological phenomenon; and it would not be erroneous to say that it resembles, for the one who experiences it, the hypnotic state, since it temporarily produces a suspension of psychical activities; it seems that he stops the course of ideas, emotions, and movements in that moment, and that his attention remains fixed on a specific point, namely on the idea or emotion suggested. [...] The brave and the eccentric bewilder, surprise, and therefore easily subjugate and prevail over the others; but, in this respect, we should also remember that in epidemics, as in any other individual psychical state, subjection and conquest through suggestion imply a privation of resistance, and therefore a form of weakness. In epidemic psychosis, undoubtedly, all the vanquished are weak.[47]

As said above, epidemic psychosis requires two main elements: a powerful idea (or emotion) expressed by some eccentric and charismatic people, and the predisposition to receive this idea, such as mental or physical vulnerability. Sergi does not hesitate to call this predisposition a *weakness*.[48] Indeed, less-educated and needy individuals are more likely to surrender to the power of suggestion, since their minds are

---

46   *Ibid.*, pp. 137–38.
47   *Ibid.*, p. 140.
48   The nexus suggestion-weakness was typical of Charcot's reflection — according to which hypnotic suggestion required a congenital vulnerability (*e.g.*, hysteria) in order to take effect —, as well as of Pierre Janet's idea of psychological automatism (originated by a state of *faiblesse psychologique*). Although Sergi does not explicitly reference these positions, his proximity to them is rather patent. Another crucial reference seems to be Hippolyte Bernheim's conception of suggestion as a universal psychological law — proper to all human beings, not only to psychiatric patients. See, Henri F. Ellenberger, *The Discovery of the Unconscious: The History and Evolution of Dynamic Psychiatry* (New York: Basic Books, 1970).

prone to unconditionally embrace new ideas — especially if these ideas appear to them as a promise of redemption or future happiness. Their naivety is also responsible for the state of bewilderment which follows the suggestion: once the course of their ideas, emotions, and movements is arrested, their attention starts to focus on a single idea, which becomes the main driver of their lives. It is a state of complete absorption, resulting in the annihilation of every personal and individual tendency.

In addition, the forms of epidemic psychosis can be manifold. In the cult of Flagellants, psychological contagion concerned ideas, emotions, and movements. Many people, understanding the Black Death to be a divine punishment, started thinking that only abnegation could mitigate God's anger. Moved by this strong conviction and influenced by the powerful emotion derived from the sight of the Flagellants, they embraced the religious ideas of the latter and resorted in turn to self-punishment. Unlike this form of psychosis, in the same period the so-called dancing mania (*mania di danzare*) only entailed a motor contagion: as Sergi recalls, it seems that in this epidemic the mere sight of a dance, performed by people allegedly struck by a sort of epileptic attack, instantly produced in those who witnessed the dance the same motor disorder. This strange epidemic is also at the origin of that well-known Italian dance called *tarantismo*.[49]

But, alongside these historical and exceptional events, what is interesting in Sergi's account is that epidemic psychosis is really a wide-ranging diagnostic category. As he states, "many social and religious revolutions took place due to epidemic psychosis".[50] Human history is thus constantly marked by psychological contagions. They are the powerful drivers of history. This means that, although Sergi devotes the majority of his study to the negative effects of epidemic psychosis, he tends nevertheless to conceive it as the qualifying feature of human interactions. As we have seen, indeed, epidemic psychosis is nothing but the pathological intensification of a normal and physiological phenomenon: suggestion. When suggestion reaches large numbers of people, it becomes epidemic. Through these concepts, it is thus possible to give a satisfactory account of what has happened in the history of humanity. And perhaps, even of what is occurring in the present day.

---

49   Sergi, *Per l'educazione del carattere*, pp. 142–43.
50   *Ibid.*, p. 144.

4. *Conclusions*

Sergi's analysis on suggestion and epidemic psychosis, beyond its interest for the historians of psychology and philosophy, could provide useful insights for the understanding of some psychological outcomes of the COVID-19 pandemic. Following Sergi's reflection, it is possible to acknowledge that what we have been facing so far are two powerful forms of contagion: one relevant for the medical diagnostics and treatment, the other relevant for the psychologist. These forms are tightly bound together, and almost indiscernible, since the latter originates from the fear and disorientation produced by the former. With the outbreak of the pandemic, a more subtle — but still insidious — contagion has spread on a global scale. Although the term "psychosis" only applies to actual mental disorders and psychiatric diseases, the idea of psychological contagion helps to explain the emergence of collective behaviors and beliefs. Powerful feelings, such as those experienced during the pandemic, can undoubtedly weaken our judgment, making us vulnerable to the influence of external suggestion. Indeed, what is said by the group is often accepted without reservation — similarly to the hypnotized who accept the orders of the hypnotist. Now, suggestion does not explain everything: even in the most complex and fearful situations, our individuality is not completely lost or absorbed in the group's will. Nevertheless, this concept helps to understand at least some psychological automatisms occurring during challenging times or upsetting events. To be dragged by the group is something that can be easily experienced on various occasions, especially when the emotional sphere takes over the conscious and intellectual one.

More interesting is probably the notion of epidemic psychosis, which can be fruitfully employed to enlighten some deviant behaviors concerning mass phenomena, that arise in correspondence to the pandemic's recrudescence. The spread of negationist movements and conspiracy theories is a case in point. Indeed, following Sergi's theory, the adhesion to non-conformist ideas can in turn be considered a form of homologation, since it is an expression of the universal law of suggestion. Although negationists and conspiracy enthusiasts claim to be free from any external conditioning or influence, they are subjected like everyone else to suggestion. Only, in this case, the suggestion received is more powerful, because it produces not only a psychological contagion, but an actual psychosis. Faced with unforeseen, unintelligible and frightening events, the search for an uncanonical way to cope with the problem is sometimes seen, by some individuals, as the only means for liberation and salvation.

Paradoxically as it is, in the era of social distancing and lockdowns, the group seems to have exerted more influence on the individual than ever. That amounts to say that social isolation does not necessarily mean psychological independence from others. What emerges from Sergi's reflection is that to belong to a group is something deeply rooted in human nature, to the point that even when social relations are limited or forbidden, some invisible threads continue to keep people in relation to each other. The boundaries between individuality and collectivity are often illusory. Also from a psychological viewpoint, it is hard to define the contours of one person's identity. That is why Sergi repeatedly reminds us that "psychic life is collective, not individual".[51]

---

51   *Ibid.*, p. 134.

Miriam Aiello, Massimo Marraffa

'THE HABITS WE ARE'[1]
The Second Nature of the Mind and Its Defences against Crisis

1. Introduction. Habits and the self

Along with the disruption of the physiology of individual and social habits, the ongoing coronavirus pandemic brings to the world population a variety of symptoms of psychological suffering and distress: important international agencies warn about the increased anxiety, anger, fear, and loss of self-efficacy.[2] The global reach and the cross-cultural transversality of this phenomenon make urgent to discuss the relationship between habits, psychological well-being and the experience of crisis from a psychological perspective.

In this contribution we address this issue through the thesis of the *defensiveness* of the self. By means of a combination of this idea with the classical philosophical figure of 'second nature' and with other categories drawn from cognitive sciences, from the psychodynamic tradition and from ethnological inquiry, it is possible to determine a stronger relation between habitual practices, the construction of the self and the experience of psychological security and insecurity.

Habits are ubiquitous phenomena that significantly affect and drive our practical, moral, epistemic and cognitive life, and that perhaps are an essential presupposition of it. Though philosophy has long neglected the study of habits, it has branched out into a fully legitimate philosophical object of inquiry within the last decade.[3]

---

1   Although this work has been conceived and written by both authors in all its parts, paragraphs 1-2 are to be attributed to Miriam Aiello, paragraphs 3-4 to Massimo Marraffa.

2   'Mental health is at the core of our humanity. It enables us to lead rich and fulfilling lives and to participate in our communities. But the COVID-19 virus is not only attacking our physical health; it is also increasing psychological suffering' (UN Secretary-General António Guterres, 13/05/2020).

3   Cf. Tom Sparrow, and Adam Hutchinson, eds., *A History of Habit. From Aristotle to Bourdieu* (Lanham: Lexington Books, 2013); Clare Carlisle, *On Habit* (New

Unfortunately, the multiple manifestations and ubiquity of habits seem to undermine the possibility of a fruitful integration of philosophical and scientific analyses, since a scientific assessment entails a wide set of distinctions and definitions of the different kinds of mechanisms that underlie (or co-occur with) different kinds of habitual behaviours,[4] which might be overlooked by a general and merely conceptual philosophical discourse.

While we keep such a difficulty into account, we nevertheless believe that both the philosophical and the psychological-scientific approach to habits bear some advantages. Thus, we sketch a possible way forward for combining the two, by conceiving of habits and of our experience of subjectivity as particular instances of a more general experience that accompanies psychological, cultural, and social experience: that of 'second nature'.

As we shall see, when examined through the lens of second nature, habitual practices and structures of personal certainty (such as psychological self-consciousness and personal identity) exhibit a number of similar features and functions, which should not lead us, however, to ignore their differences.

One might argue that there are at least two different ways of addressing the issue regarding the link between habits and psychological life. The first way, which relies on the substantialist intuitions of folk psychology, views psychological life as a *presupposition* of the development of habits, and the latter as 'belonging' to the subject who develops them: a conscious subject is assumed as the bearer of habits. According to the second way, we should rather ask to what extent, and in which sense, psychological life itself has a 'second-natural' and/or 'habitual' structure.

In §2, we will suggest that there are some similarities between the 'habits we have' and the 'habits we are', based on the idea of a 'second nature of the mind' (or of mind as second nature). We will argue that the relation between unconscious cognitive processes and self-consciousness can be regarded as a relation between a 'first' and a 'second' nature. Such a claim is coherent with the results of the cognitive sciences and of

---

York: Routledge, 2014); Marco Piazza, *L'antagonista necessario. La filosofia francese dell'abitudine da Montaigne a Bergson* (Milan: Mimesis, 2015); Marco Piazza, *Creature dell'abitudine: abito, costume, seconda natura da Aristotele alle scienze cognitive* (Bologna: Il Mulino, 2018).

4   E.g., we can see that the development of habits concerns and overlaps at least the notions of script, plan, schema, skill, behavioural pattern, as well as those of compulsion and addiction on the pathological side.

contextualistic and systemic perspectives on the genesis of selfhood, which also account for our deceptive folk intuition regarding the primitiveness of self-consciousness.

In §3, we will underline the defensive function of both habits and the self. Drawing on Dan McAdams' theory of narrative identity and his definition of the self as a selfing process, we will argue that the narrative construction of identity takes shape according to a fundamental egological need: that is, the primal need to subsist subjectively and, thereby, to face the lack of a metaphysical guarantee of the unity of the mind. In the practical sphere, this defensive and precarious construction is embedded in a network of activities and processes aimed at defending the self-image and at displaying a socially recognized identity. We will also show how a subject's ordinary experience of the world presupposes an objectual and interpersonal environment marked with emotional and evaluative connotations, which organize an ordered, meaningful and domestic reality, whereby not only practical habits, but also prejudices and self-deceptive uses of causal attribution play a protective role.

In the conclusive remarks (§4), we will claim that every disruption of habits, as it dismantles the more superficial layers of the construction of reality, brings to the fore the selfing process and its defensive functions. We will also outline a spectrum of four combinations of defensive endowments according to their capacity to provide the subject with ontological security. We will then argue that, although habits and the selfing activity share a defensive function against the threat of disintegration, the key-role in providing effective protection of the unity of the mind and the meaningfulness of the experience pertains to the degree of psychological self-integration. Lastly, examining the issue of crisis from the standpoint of the interaction between individual and social mechanisms of defence, we will outline a difference between the (mainly social) way of coping with crisis and disruption in pre-literate or in traditional societies, and the (mainly individual) way promoted by late-modern societies.

2. The 'second natural' life of the mind

Second nature is a long-lasting philosopheme in Western tradition. From Aristotle to Hegel, from Montaigne to McDowell, several philosophers put forth the idea that culture (broadly speaking) endows human animals with a set of properties that are not natural. Moreover, these thinkers seem to suggest that cultural properties take root in the natural properties that regulate human biological existence, so that they are in fact, from a 'phenomenal' perspective, mutually inseparable[5]. Drawing on this tradition, we can hypothesize that second nature is a peculiar kind of nature *impressed upon* a first nature. 'First' nature is a set of natural kinds that depend on laws of nature, irrespective of human knowledge, perception, action, and interest.[6] By contrast, second nature refers to the cultural and historical environment, including any kind of cultural activities, artefacts, or institutions actively shaped by the human species according to its practical interests.

Second nature implies an analogical relation to *first* nature, which is worth unravelling. The ordinal adjective 'second' denotes something that comes both 'after' and 'above' something else that, in turn, comes 'before' and 'below', and that is therefore 'first' from a chronological, logical, and ontological point of view. The first-natural order constitutes, at least to a certain extent, a model for the second-natural level. The definition of culture as second nature entails the idea that culture is somehow akin or *commeasurable to nature*, in that a) it displays the same given and pre-reflexive character as first nature; and b) it affects human conduct as if it had the same causal power of a natural law. When we say that habits, myths, rites, customs, laws, traditions, aesthetic forms, etc., are 'second nature', we of course mean, on the one hand, that these entities are not strictly natural, for they were *produced* by actions of human individuals and groups; but on the other hand, we also mean that these entities influence and shape human behaviour in a seemingly unquestionable manner, which resembles the way natural laws determine natural phenomena.

Based on the previous remarks, we should then try to verify if the relation between the functional structure of the mind as described by cognitive science and the folk image of mental life can be fruitfully described in terms of a relation between first and second nature. More specifically, we should assess whether it is possible to identify in our mental life any structures which, though having a natural implementation, are fostered by cultural and social stimulations. Or, put another way, whether second nature can

---

5   Some authors claim that the phenomenal conflation is also a substantive conflation, so that once the natural dimension has been completely merged with the cultural one, it would be no longer identifiable as self-standing. We argue that such a view should be rejected, insofar as it hinders any attempt to give a naturalistic account of mental phenomena.

6   Alexander Bird, and Emma Tobin, 'Natural Kinds', in *The Stanford Encyclopedia of Philosophy (Spring 2018 Edition)*, ed. by Edward N. Zalta, <https://plato.stanford.edu/archives/spr2018/entries/natural-kinds/> (last access: November 14th, 2021).

express the relationship between the scientific and the manifest image of the mind, between third person-descriptions and first person-experience.[7] Before proceeding further, we would like to make clear that the essential core of this thesis is not new: the idea that some inferential habit lies at the basis of our intuition of subjectivity was first set forth in a fully-fledged version in Hume's *Treatise*,[8] and more recently by his most prominent contemporary epigone, Dennett,[9] who explains the rise of consciousness in our ancestors in terms of habits of self-stimulation.

A first reason why speaking of a 'second nature of the mind' may be appropriate has something to do with the fact that most contemporary research in the cognitive sciences conceives of consciousness as a *derived and non-primary* phenomenon.

The cognitive sciences systematically invoke explanations of behavior in which mental processes are unconscious operations on as much rigorously unconscious representational states; and indeed, the theoretical appeal to the 'cognitive' (or 'computational') unconscious has been so accentuated that it can be maintained that in the present day the unconscious reigns over our whole mental existence. This approach to the mental – Fodor[10] reminds us – would have not been possible in the pre-Freudian conceptual universe, where an inextricable link between consciousness and intentionality was in force. It is to Freud's credit that he challenged this nexus; for he gave plausibility to the idea that the explanation of behavior might require the postulation of intentional *but* unconscious mental states. An idea that Fodor concludes has been amply vindicated, most especially in Chomskian linguistics and in cognitive psychology.

However, this historical note needs to be rectified: the cognitive sciences have not simply vindicated Freud but have gone far beyond. In fact, consciousness is taken by Freud as a self-evident, primary quality of the mind, although it is then criticized and 'downsized' in comparison to the traditional idealistic view; Freud's notion of the unconscious is parasitic to this concept of consciousness.[11] On the other hand, in Freudian

---

7   Cf. Gerald M. Edelman, *Second nature. Brain science and human knowledge* (New Heaven: Yale University Press, 2006).

8   David Hume, *A Treatise of Human Nature* (Oxford: Oxford University Press, 2000).

9   Daniel C. Dennett, *Consciousness explained* (Boston: Little Brown, 1991).

10   Jerry A. Fodor, 'Too hard for our kind of mind?', *London Review of Books*, 13, 12 (1991).

11   Giovanni Jervis, 'The unconscious', in *Cartographies of the mind*, ed. by Massimo Marraffa, Mario De Caro and Francesco Ferretti (Berlin: Springer, 2007), 147–58 (p. 152).

psychoanalysis the idea of the mind is still dominated by the model of the conscious elaboration of choices, and within it, the unconscious plays its tricks here and there, but nothing more. In short, Freud remains a Cartesian.

Things are very different in the case of the cognitive sciences, where the mind is conceived as a process of construction and transformation of representations, and a mental representation is an explanatory hypothesis in a computational theory of cognition.[12] It is a structure of information (somehow encoded in the brain), which is individuated exclusively in terms of intra-theoretical functional criteria, in which the phenomenological aspects play no role whatsoever.

As a result, the cognitive sciences open the conceptual space to build a consciousness-independent conception of the unconscious. As Dennett puts it, first one develops a theory of intentionality that is independent of and more fundamental than consciousness; a theory that treats equally any form of unconscious representational mentality "in brains, in computers, in evolution's 'recognition' of properties of selected designs".[13] One can then proceed to work out a theory of consciousness on that foundation. In this perspective, consciousness is an advanced or derived mental phenomenon and not, as Descartes wanted, the foundation of all mental life. In short, 'first intentionality, then consciousness'.[14]

In viewing consciousness no longer as something that explains, but rather as something that is to be explained, analyzed, and dismantled, the cognitive sciences amend the Freudian thought on the basis of Darwinian naturalism. Differently from Freud's introspective account of the unconscious, the cognitive sciences capitalize on Darwin's anti-idealistic methodological lesson and proceed *bottom-up*, attempting to reconstruct how the complex psychological functions underlying the adult self-conscious mind evolve from the more basic ones.[15]

---

12   Robert Cummins, *Representations, targets and attitudes* (Cambridge, MA: MIT Press, 1997).
13   Dennett, p. 66.
14   *Ibid.*
15   This bottom-up perspective coincides with what Piaget called "decentration of the subject" (Giovanni Jervis, *Fondamenti di psicologia dinamica*, Milan: Feltrinelli, 1993, p. 243). In its disclosing the non-primary but derived, constructed, and partial character of self-consciousness, the cognitive sciences' bottom-up approach can be regarded as an *anti-phenomenology*, i.e., a critique of the subject, of its alleged givenness (Giovanni Jervis, *La psicoanalisi come esercizio critico*, Milan: Garzanti, 1989, p. 36). The term "anti-phenomenology" is used by Paul Ricoeur to define psychoanalysis: the latter, he writes, is "an antiphenomenology which requires, not the reduction *to* consciousness, but the reduction *of*

This developmental approach to the self does not appeal to our introspective self-knowledge, but rather to the results of investigations into the gradual construction of human self-awareness. In this perspective, the study of the 0–1-year-old infant's subjectivity should follow the example of the study of animal subjectivity, where cogent evidence can be found of very complex inter-individual behavioral dynamics that are produced by conscious (but not self-conscious) activities of representation. Starting from the automatic and pre-reflexive forming representations of the external world ('object consciousness'), the human neurocognitive system produces, over a period of about 15-18-24 months, a representation of the body as a whole: a *bodily* self.[16] Then an introspective experiential space is constructed, endowing the subject with a psychological self-consciousness. This is the result of the 'affectivation' of bodily reflexivity first,[17] and then of turning upon oneself a collection of other-directed social-cognitive abilities subserved by two early-developing neurocomputational systems: one underlying the psychological reasoning or "mindreading", the other underpinning sociomoral reasoning.[18] Finally, with the development of autobiographical memory and autobiographical reasoning, psychological self-consciousness evolves in the ability to construct a self-narrative as a layer of personality.[19]

This developmental framework for conceptualizing the self is also a psychodynamic and socio-cognitive framework, avoiding an overly reductionist approach that would explain everything in terms of bottom-up

---

cosciousness" (Paul Ricoeur, *The Conflict of Interpretations: Essays in Hermeneutics*, ed. by Don Hide, trans. by Kathleen McLaughlin et al., London: The Athlone Press, 1989, p. 237). However, as we have just seen, Freud's inquiry into the unconscious starts from a consciousness taken as a given fact; this makes psychoanalysis a dialectical variant of phenomenology. In contrast, the cognitive sciences, fortified by a consciousness-independent concept of intentionality, have full right to qualify as an anti-phenomenology.

16   Michael Lewis and Jeanne Brooks-Gunn, *Social cognition and the acquisition of self* (New York: Plenum Press, 1979).

17   Peter Fonagy, and others, *Affect regulation, mentalization, and the development of the self* (London: Other Press, 2002).

18   Melody Buyukozer Dawkins, and others, 'Early moral cognition: a principle-based approach', in *The cognitive neurosciences*, ed. by David Poeppel, George R. Mangun and Michael S. Gazzaniga (Cambridge, MA: The MIT Press, 2020), 7–16.

19   Dan P. McAdams, *The art and science of personality development* (New York-London: Guilford Press, 2016); Tilmann Habermas, and Christin Köber, 'Autobiographical reasoning in life narratives buffers the effect of biographical disruptions on the sense of self- continuity', *Memory*, 23, 5 (2015), 664–74.

neurocognitive mechanisms. This is achieved through a *contextualist* and *systemic* perspective, where the individual's psychological problems are investigated by putting them in the inter-individual and social context in which they arise and obtain meaning. This systemic approach to the study of relationality is at the heart of the theory of object relations and attachment theory – as Donald Winnicott puts it, what makes sense is not considering the infant in itself, but the mother-infant dyad. From Bowlby's study of anaclitic depression in abandoned children to the more recent hypothesis on disorganized attachment as an etiological factor of borderline personality disorder, attachment theory has strongly emphasized the role of caring social relationships for the development of a structure of personality and a sense of self marked by ontological security. This psychodynamic tradition suggests that, far from being the fundament of human mindedness, self-consciousness and the self are rather an ontogenetical achievement that needs a social and emotive relationship in order to be fulfilled.

This naturalistic, bottom-up, and systemic-relational framework offers further reasons to suggest the analogical definition of the self as a second-natural habit. Such a habit can be thought of as a 'habit we are', in that a) it cannot be attributed to an independent and previously existing self, but rather coincides with the very formation of the self. It can be conceived as second-natural, for it b) stems from first-natural processes; c) is endowed with nature-like causal power; and d) appears to us as a natural given – we fall prey, so to speak, to a 'natural idealistic self-deception'.[20]

3. *The defensive life of the mind*

We have so far suggested that there is a conceptual *continuum*, or at least a 'family resemblance', between 'the habits we have' and 'the habits we are', in that they share a 'second-natural' fundament. We will now argue that they also share a similar *defensive* function. However, it should be stressed that these similarities do not entail overlapping or interchangeability: the two kinds of habit are not one and the same, and the second nature of the mind is not a habit in the ordinary sense. There are, indeed, two connected asymmetries concerning the relationship between the self and the practical habits.

---

20   Giovanni Jervis, *Il mito dell'interiorità*, ed. by Gilberto Corbellini and Massimo Marraffa (Turin: Bollati Boringhieri, 2011), p. 198.

(1) The building process of psychological self-consciousness and self-identity is far more complex than the acquisition of a habit, which relies on association patterns and can take place at different developmental stages. On the contrary, as we have seen, the rise of a full-fledged self-consciousness and of a sense of selfhood require not only bodily self-awareness and emotional scaffolding, but also and more importantly, autobiographical memory and some peculiar narrative abilities.

A continuous effort of integration is needed for the development of personal identity: the subject constantly unifies self-referred pieces of experience and spins them into a narrative web which has *the format of a life-story*.

Over the last three decades Dan McAdams has developed a life-story model of identity at the interface of personality psychology, life-span developmental studies, and cultural psychology. Making a synthesis of William James' theory of duplex self, Erik Erikson's view of identity, and Henry Murray's research program on the Study of Lives, McAdams[21] proposed a theory of identity development in which narrative identity is seen as a social-affective-cognitive structure designed to provide that sense of temporal sameness and continuity that Erikson thought to be a defining feature of identity.[22]

Within McAdams' theoretical framework, narrative identity is the internalized and evolving story of the self which integrates the reconstructed past and the imagined future to provide life with some degree of unity, purpose, and meaning. This process of integration is construed in terms of James's classic theory of the self as constituted by the couple <I, Me>. McAdams interprets James as arguing that the self-as-I (the self as a subject) is not "the inner psychological entity that is the center or subject of a person's experience".[23] The I is rather a *process*; "I" does not refer to a noun but to a *verb*: "it might be called 'selfing' or 'I-ing', the fundamental

21 Dan P. McAdams, *Power, intimacy, and the life story: Personological inquiries into identity* (Homewood, IL: Dorsey Press, 1985).

22 Around the same time, Katherine Nelson (ed., *Narratives from the crib*, Cambridge, MA: Harvard University Press, 1989) proposed a theory of early narrative development that has since been associated to McAdams' theory. See for references: Kate C. McLean, and Moin Syed (2015), 'The field of identity development needs an identity', in *The Oxford handbook of identity development*, ed. by Idd. (Oxford-New York: Oxford University Press, 2015), 1–10 (p. 2).

23 Mark R. Leary, and June P. Tangney, eds., *Handbook of self and identity* (New York: The Guilford Press, 2012), p. 5.

process of making a self out of experience".[24] By contrast, James' self-as-Me (the self as object) is "the primary product of the selfing process"; it is "the self that selfing makes".[25] The Me exists as an evolving collection of self-attributions (James' material, social and psychological selves) which originate from the I-ing process. It is "the making of the Me that constitutes what the I fundamentally is".[26]

Thus, in contrast to those philosophical views that take self-consciousness as a basic modality of consciousness, a primary and simple 'knowing of being-there'[27], James defines self-consciousness in terms of *identity*: it is a knowing of being-there *in a certain way*, a self-describing, an identity forming, which is "a unifying, integrative, synthesizing process".[28] So interpreted, James' theory of the self anticipates a number of theories in developmental and personality psychology that have made appeal to a general organismic process for integrating subjective experience. Ryan[29] mentions Heinz Werner's orthogenetic principle, Jean Piaget's organization, and Carl Gustav Jung's individuation; despite all their differences, these constructs share the idea that human experience tends

---

24   Dan P. McAdams, 'Personality, modernity, and the storied self: A contemporary framework for studying persons', *Psychological Inquiry*, 7 (1996), 295–321 (p. 302).

25   McAdams, 'Personality, modernity, and the storied self: A contemporary framework for studying persons'.

26   Dan P. McAdams, and Keith S. Cox, 'Self and identity across the life span', in *The Handbook of Life-Span Development*, ed. by Richard M. Lerner (New York: Wiley, 2010), II, 158–207 (p. 162).

27   The main reference here is to what Kant asserts in a famous passage of the first *Critique*. As is well known, Kant agrees with Hume that the empirical apperception "can give us no constant or enduring self in the flow of inner appearances" (Immanuel Kant, *Critique of pure reason*, Cambridge: Cambridge University Press, 1998, p. 232, A 107). Yet, he thinks that one may shift from the analysis level of psychological experience to that of transcendental arguing, and here posits a pure apperception: "I am conscious of myself, not as I appear to myself, nor as I am in myself, but only that I am", he writes in the first *Critique* (B157); in B158 he adds that "[t]he consciousness of self is [...] far from being a knowledge of the self" – i.e., the consciousness of existing is distinguished from the consciousness of existing in a certain way. Thus Kant's I think ("that accompanies all my representations") is something undetermined and void ("a something=X"), which, not unlike Descartes' cogito, lays a claim to being a *primum*.

28   Dan P. McAdams, 'The case for unity in the (post)modern self: A modest proposal', in *Self and identity. Fundamental issues*, ed. by Richard D. Ashmore and Lee Jussim (New York: Oxford University Press, 1997), 46–78 (p. 56).

29   Richard M. Ryan, 'Psychological needs and the facilitation of integrative processes', *Journal of Personality*, 63 (1995), 397–427, cit. in McAdams, 1997.

toward "a fundamental sense of unity in that human beings apprehend experience through an integrative selfing process".[30]

McAdams embeds this interpretation of James' theory of self in his framework for conceptualizing the whole person across her life span. Here narrative identity hinges on two other cognitive layers. The first consists of a small set of broad *dispositional traits* implicated in social life, which account for consistencies in behavioural style from one situation to the next and over time. The second layer consists of a wide range of *characteristic adaptations* (including goals, strivings, personal projects, values, interests, defence mechanisms, coping strategies, relational schemata) which capture more socially contextualised and motivational aspects of psychological individuality. During personality development, people's internalised and evolving life stories are layered over characteristic adaptations, which are, in turn, layered over dispositional traits. This process of layering may be *integrative*: the process of selfing may succeed in bringing traits, skills, goals, values, and experiences together into a meaningful life story.[31]

Habermas and Bluck[32] have described the social-cognitive changes that must take place in order for the adolescent to initiate the crafting of the life story that is at the heart of McAdams's theory. The life story is most completely manifested in entire life narratives as specific, but rare, linguistic products. A more frequent but only partial manifestation of the life story is what Habermas and Bluck termed 'autobiographical reasoning' which is the activity of using 'autobiographical arguments' for creating links between personal experiences and other distant parts of one's life, and to the self and its development.[33] This activity is termed "reasoning" to underscore three aspects: the constructive and interpretative nature of the

---

30   McAdams, 'The case for unity in the (post)modern self', p. 57.
31   The difficulties normal adults belonging to preliterate cultures face in conceptualizing their own psychological experience provide a significant counterfactual to this account of the rise of an inner virtual space of the mind. In these cultures, social and bodily identity are seamlessly connected, and the individuals lack a private inner psychological space in which intentions and emotions can be identified and elaborated. This absence affects both the mechanisms of causal attribution and the manifestations of mental distress. Lacking a conceptualization of their own mental sphere, preliterate subjects are prone to somatization, hysterical-dissociative phenomena, as well as to religious and magical rationalization.
32   Tilmann Habermas, and Susan Bluck, 'Getting a life: the emergence of the life story in adolescence', *Psychological Bulletin*, 126, 5 (2000), 748–69.
33   Tilmann Habermas, 'Autobiographical reasoning: Arguing and narrating from a biographical perspective', *New Directions for Child and Adolescent Development*, 131 (2011), 1–17.

activity, its cognitive and communicative nature, and its normative aspect implied by its appeal to reason and logic.[34]

Autobiographical reasoning involves four socio-cognitive capacities, creating four kinds of coherence that are decisive for the overall global coherence of life narratives: (i) the capacity to create temporal orientation by sequential structure and chronology (*temporal* coherence); (ii) the ability to think about the self in abstract terms (i.e., as embodying certain personality traits) and account for changes or developments in the self over time (*causal-motivational* coherence); (iii) the ability to summarize and interpret themes within stories and apply these to one's own life (*thematic* coherence); and (iv) having an awareness of cultural norms regarding the major milestones and events one is expected to experience during the life course.

In an influential review, Habermas and de Silveira[35] showed that a life narrative begins to emerge in middle childhood, but the coherence of this narrative (in all its dimensions) increases during adolescence. Köber, Schmiedek and Habermas[36] longitudinally extended this study to explore the development of global coherence in life narratives from childhood to adulthood. It was found that measures of temporal and causal-motivational coherence increase substantially across adolescence up to early adulthood, as does thematic coherence, which continues to develop throughout middle adulthood.

This brief overview on the narrative building of the self sheds light on the fact that the selfing process, as it requires effort to cope narratively with constantly changing pieces of experience, lacks the automaticity of habits. It should also be noted that selfing gains real causal efficacy. Unlike the

---

34   The term 'reasoning' also alludes to the Piagetian cognitive-developmental tradition, which Habermas and Bluck aim to wed to the narrative tradition. In full harmony with Piaget's constructivism (Habermas and Bluck, p. 749) describe the development of the life story in adolescence as the emergence of a new quality, the "global coherence of the life story". To convey the development of the self, up to the present, life narratives not only require the inclusion of various life events and aspects of the self, but also interpretive connections between events and self in order to create a globally coherent story. Global coherence is the narrative feature that differentiates life narratives from mere lists of unrelated memories from one's life.

35   Tilmann Habermas, and Cybèle de Silveira, 'The development of global coherence in life narratives across adolescence: Temporal, causal, and thematic aspects', *Developmental Psychology*, 44 (2008), 707–21.

36   Christin Köber, Florian Schmiedek and Tilmann Habermas, 'Characterizing lifespan development of three aspects of coherence in life narratives: a cohort-sequential study', *Developmental Psychology*, 51 (2015), 260–75.

continuously self-rewriting autobiographies of Dennett's Joycean machine, identity as a story of the self is by no means contingent and evanescent; it is *a layer of personality that represents a causal center of gravity*.

(2) The 'habits we are' are 'stronger' and structurally primary when compared to the 'habits we have', and also work as an organizational centre of practical habits. Following Pierre Bourdieu's thinking, we can say that one's habitus is not reducible to his or her habits[37]. In fact, the disruption of habits does not imply any automatic disruption of the self. The selfing process and its continuous effort of integration work at a deeper level, and function as "a centre of emanation of defensive strategies": the most inner one is probably the already mentioned autobiographical reasoning, the ability to connect in a causal and coherent fashion the events in a life-story within the autobiographical memory system. Conversely, the practical habits that make one's world domestic, meaningful, and operable, appear as more peripheral coping strategies.

Having established these pivotal differences, we can get back to the *defensive* functional ground shared by both the self and practical habits.

The self works as an 'integration machine', which requires constant narrative and creative efforts; but it is also and perhaps more radically a 'defensive machine'. That is, the self as finding oneself again as a known identity, as a feeling of biographical continuity, is a precarious acquisition, continuously constructed by the person and constantly exposed to the risk of disaggregation.[38] This precariousness is the key to understanding the defensiveness immanent to the selfing process. The need to construct and protect an identity that is valid to the greatest extent possible is rooted in the primary need to subsist subjectively, and thus to exist solidly as a describable ego, as a unitary subject. Human self-conscious subjectivity constitutes itself as a repertoire of composite psychological maneuvers, of activities that take pains to cope with its lack of ontological guarantee, constructing itself on the edge of its original "non-being", as it were.

---

37   "I say habitus also and especially *for not saying* 'habit'": Pierre Bourdieu, and Löic Wacquant, *Risposte. Per un'antropologia riflessiva* (Turin: Bollati Boringhieri, 1992), p. 90.

38   The precarious nature of the subject's self-construction is well captured by the concept of "presence" of the philosopher-anthropologist Ernesto de Martino. Presence is the finding oneself again at the center of a one's own orderly and meaningful subjective world, and hence at the center of an historical and cultural environment to which one feels to belong. But this finding oneself again is a precarious acquisition, continuously constructed by the subject and constantly exposed to the risk of the crisis (the crisis of presence).

Within this framework, defensiveness is therefore a constitutive trait of our mental life, rather than a dysfunctional one. According to Jervis,[39] the aspects of human life that involve ambiguity, self-deception, and suffering can no longer be conceived as the philosophical tradition has viewed them, namely, as the crisis of a fundamentally rational agent, temporarily overwhelmed by the perturbing influence of affects and sentiments. These aspects can now be conceived as *globally constitutive* dimensions of the mind and conduct. This gives place to a reinforcing overturning of the psychoanalytic questioning of defences: what we now have to ask ourselves is not how and why some defensive mechanisms exist, but rather if it is not the case that *all* the structures of knowledge and action around which everyday life is structured serve a defensive function.

Here, then, we grasp something that is already in Freud but which the Cartesian framework of instinctual drives prevented him from articulating fully: the defensive processes are much more than bulwarks against anxieties and insecurities that perturb the order of our inner life; they are the primary instruments for establishing order in the mind; they are the very structure of the mind – the Freudian ego itself is a defense.

In this theoretical framework, dynamic psychology joins forces with interpersonal and social psychology. The defense of self-image (closely linked to the self-defensive use of causal attribution), the social attitudes in general and the stereotypes and prejudices in particular, and the rationalizing handling of cognitive dissonance are the building blocks of an interpersonal and social reality packed with systematic errors or, as Freud would have put it, interested self-deceptions. All of these structures of self-deception are defensive constructions that spring from mental operations in which the cognitive aspect cannot be separated from the affective. To illustrate, we briefly focus on the construct of prejudice.

'Knowing' – as well as 'making sense' – is primarily a pragmatic matter, a 'knowing how to do things'. In the context of everyday life an object makes sense for me, and it is known by me, because I place it in a pragmatic context, insofar as I consider it within a repertoire of competences: I have done something with this object in the past and I can do something with it in the future. But there is inherent in the very idea of 'knowing how to do' an organization of the world according to differentiations and hierarchies. All of us, in forming more or less complex behavioral patterns, act according to gradients of involvement and interest. Basically, we assign different

---

39   Jervis, *Fondamenti di psicologia dinamica*.

'values' to single objects and to different aspects of our behavior itself.[40] The panorama of reality takes shape then in accordance with our interests for objects, viz. according to the value that we assign to the surroundings:

> Clusters, hierarchies of values arise; the various areas of reality are on different grades of importance. The 'nearer' scenarios are those that we are more interested in, and are easily the object of our 'positive' planning; the more 'distant' scenarios are those we are less interested in; they are less differentiated in their internal details, and can more easily appear to be extraneous or even hostile. These variables come to be organized in the first place according to the phenomenological category of 'domesticity', or 'familiarity'. All of us tend to make a spontaneous separation between, on the one hand, what is 'internal' to a limited, 'domestic' social world, and hence 'good' and 'reassuring', and where we find, as it were, a proximal panorama of guaranteed values; and, on the other end, what is 'external', 'alien', which we are less interested in, whose guaranteed value is lower, and where objects and events can take on negative tones.[41]

This way of organizing reality, and of situating ourselves at its center, is a primary way of 'establishing order', which has clear affinities with some basic structuring categories such as 'before-after', 'high-low', and above all, in our case, 'inner-outer' and 'near-distant'. The phenomenological category of domesticity refers to the experience of the world-environment as structured according to criteria of distance and controllability. This is a primarily cognitive operation, but one which is nevertheless linked to the attribution of emotional-evaluative connotations in conformity with the so-called 'primary affects', i.e., according to a basic alternative of our dispositional orientation toward reality that sharply distinguishes

---

40 'Values' are to be understood here as simple differences of importance, i.e., of priority, in the context of the general theme of adaptation. There is an objectivity in the gradients of value in specific contexts. In the cycle of everyday activities, animals organize their behavior as a function of a limited series of general interests ('evolutionary values') such as predator defense, foraging, defense of rank in group hierarchy, and reproduction: each of these general needs dominates over specific behavioral patterns which from time to time are a higher priority than others, i.e., literally 'they come before' insofar as they 'have more value', alternating with each other at the top of the agenda of 'the things to do'. In ethology, behavioral priorities can be quantified by means of game theory. See John Maynard-Smith, *Evolution and the theory of games* (Cambridge: Cambridge University Press, 1982).

41 Jervis, *Fondamenti di psicologia dinamica*, p. 331, transl. ours.

pleasantness and unpleasantness, friend and foe, and thereby coming closer and going away, accepting and rejecting, encompassing and expelling.[42]

In animals the world tends to get organized in accordance with the category of territoriality; we find, in ways that are different depending on the species, the den as the most protected shelter, and more outwardly a 'possession zone', an 'exploratory zone', and so on. In children the 'domestic space' is linked to the presence of the primary attachment figure: the possibility of exploring, leaving the 'protection zone', appears to be proportional to the level of reassurance provided by the caregiver.[43] In adults the difficulty of leaving the 'domestic zone' has been called 'territorial anguish' by De Martino,[44] and viewed by the philosopher-ethnologist as one of the two main parameters of the feeling of being in crisis: the spatial or geographic parameter as opposed to the temporal one.

This brings us to prejudice, because its psychological dynamic belongs precisely to that way of organizing reality and placing ourselves at its center that we have just been sketching. That is, the dynamics of prejudice are part and parcel of the ways in which we spontaneously systematize the material or social reality according to categories of relevance and gradients of approval and disapproval. The peculiarity of prejudice consists in the fact that, whereas in most of our basic attitudes (of liking, curiosity, identification, wish, disposition to the affective bond, etc.) there is a ('positive') tendency to approach the object. In prejudice we find the opposite tendency, to reject the object, which results in a refusal to know it. Now, according to the social identity theory, feeling a member of the ingroup is closely linked to stigmatizing the outgroup members as treacherous and different.[45] As a result, expressing the prejudice (i.e. the stereotype) at the moment in which it brings discredit on 'the others', accomplishes the defensive (self-apologetic) function of enhancing our self-image, providing us with a collective identity (a sense of community), which is also a certificate of nobility that 'the others' do not possess. Feeling comfortably part of a 'valid' community causes us to believe in our

---

42   See the circumplex model of affect in James A. Russell, 'A circumplex model of affect', *Journal of Personality and Social Psychology*, 39 (1980), 1161–78.

43   Cf. Mary S. Ainsworth, and others, *Patterns of attachment: A psychological study of the strange situation* (Oxford: Lawrence Erlbaum, 1978).

44   Ernesto De Martino, 'Angoscia territoriale e riscatto culturale nel mito Achilpa delle origini', *Studi e Materiali di Storia delle religioni*, 23 (1951-52), 51–66.

45   Cf., e.g., Henri Tajfel, and John C. Turner, 'The social identity theory of intergroup behavior', in *Psychology of intergroup relations*, ed. by Stephen Worchel and William L. Austin (Chicago: Nelson-Hall, 1986), 7–24.

inner validity. The biasing aspect of prejudice can thus be ascribed to the very ways in which ordinary knowledge constitutes itself.

4. Conclusions. The re-domestication of the world and the frail self

If we reassess the relation between habits and selfhood in light of the previous remarks, we can argue that the system of habits tends to overshadow the defensiveness of the self. This means that whenever habits crack, this defensiveness emerges more clearly. The disruption of habits weakens the domestic relationship with the world, exposes the frailty of the self and calls upon it to buffer the disruption as best as it can. While in normal conditions the self-memory system is enough to guarantee biographical continuity (in that it provides for the continuity of identity through the continuous adjustment of past self-representations to present self-representations[46] – in case of disrupting events or conditions (like in grief and mourning), autobiographical reasoning steps in and provides a more powerful buffering effect.[47] The disruption of habits compels the subject to reorganize and refurbish its defensive repertoire, i.e., to re-narrate himself against ontological insecurity, and to figure out new habits that make the world familiar again. The COVID-19 pandemic has displayed many social and individual practices of re-domestication of the world and of the interpersonal space (cf. Stefano De Matteis' contribution in this volume). Of course, it has also caused severe crisis to some individuals, especially the most fragile. The 'habits we are' and their degree of self-integration play a more structural role in coping with crisis than practical habits, which represent – as we have argued – second-order coping mechanisms.[48] We can try to distinguish four macro-categories of individuals whose protective mechanisms range from the higher degree of ontological security to the lower one:

1. Highly-integrated selves and functioning habits
2. Highly-integrated selves and disrupted habits
3. Weakly-integrated selves and functioning habits
4. Weakly-integrated selves and disrupted habits

---

46   Martin A. Conway, 'Memory and the self', *Journal of Memory and Language*, 53, 4 (2005), 594–628.
47   Köber, Schmiedek and Habermas.
48   We can place habits at the level of characteristic adaptations, the second layer of McAdams' personological model.

This outline refers to two different kinds of individuals in conditions of biographical continuity (case 1 and 3) and in disrupting circumstances (case 2 and 4). It may be supposed that individuals belonging to these different clusters would display different attitudes and patterns of reaction in coping with crisis as well as different degrees of ontological security, in accordance with their different combinations of defensive endowments. It stands to reason that individuals belonging to cluster 4, who more than others lack defensive tools, would experience the lowest degree of ontological security and less effective ability to manage with abnormal experiences. Determining the degree of ontological security of clusters 2 and 3 might seem more puzzling: but, again, with reference to McAdams' model (§2), it is more reasonable to think that highly integrated selves in conditions of biographical disruption would have the narrative and motivational resources to endogenously rearrange their psychological continuity and to renovate their characteristic adaptations successfully, whereas the weakly integrated selves, even in case of biographical continuity, would obtain an exogenous psychological balance and sense of unity mainly through the provisional accordance of external conditions and practical habits. This spectrum could be *per se* a useful tool to account for the differentiated outcomes in coping with crisis. However, it may benefit from a theoretical integration, which we have only outlined, with cultural anthropology and with De Martino's[49] reflections about psychopathological and cultural apocalypses. This further addition stresses the importance to analyse the issue of the crisis also in the light of the dialectic between individual and social mechanisms of defence.

A number of objections could be raised against the universalization of the modern and western structure of subjectivity and of its strategies for coping with crisis. However, there is some evidence for claiming that the ego dissolution – as the most extreme form of loss of unity of the mind – is a transhistorical and transcultural phenomenon. De Martino's work shows how, in preliterate cultures, the social group provides mythical-ritual protocols that accompany the suffering subject into a socially guided and controlled form of loss of presence that also contains a promise of full restoration of presence and leads to a strengthening of social bonds. In these societies, the crisis of presence is a social fact, and the social order offers a protective belt, so to say, to manage it. This is the reason why, according to De Martino, even in the worst and most socially dangerous scenario, that

---

49   Ernesto De Martino, *La fine del mondo. Contributo all'analisi delle apocalissi culturali* (Turin: Einaudi, 2019).

of a cultural apocalypse, the prognosis of a crisis of presence is favourable as long as the mythical-ritual protocols are accepted and trusted. But what happens in late modern societies? A well-established sociological tradition has asserted that contemporary western societies are post-traditional, disenchanted and secularized orders, and that individuals therein should be seen as responsible and creative agents who take on the risk of existence.[50] In this framework, the protection and restoration of presence is mostly an individual, not social, fact and task. It is true, as Bourdieu[51] argued, that society continues to foster some administered forms of self-description that provides for some very weak forms of self-unification, which nonetheless seem to be insufficient for coping with extraordinary disruptions. The failure of a life project often leads to a pathological outcome, as in the case of addictions.[52] Here the prognosis, as De Martino[53] already observed for the case of psychopathological apocalypse, is less auspicious and riskier.

And yet we should note in De Martino as well an ambivalence toward the capacity of the mythical-ritual techniques to really play a role in the self-protection of presence. On one hand, "as a progressivist, a socialist, and an expert on the problems of southern Italy", De Martino could not miss that some aspects of southern Italian culture "were imprisonment, psychological regression, a hindrance in the way of progress and of the emancipation of the masses";[54] he could not be unaware of the fact that the ritual device, a collective and cultural phenomenon, "keeps in itself a trace, a remnant of the individual and pre-cultural neurotic compulsion".[55] On the other hand, his historicism, and his curiosity for the possible aspects of truth in the magical-religious traditions, led him to emphasize "the autonomy, dignity, and functionality of ritual mechanisms, at the expense of any suspicion about them".[56] This, for example, in the context of the

---

50   Antony Giddens, *Modernity and self-identity* (Cambridge: Polity Press, 1991).

51   Pierre Bourdieu, 'L'illusion biographique', *Actes de la Recherche en Sciences Sociales*, 62-63 (1986), 69–70.

52   Antony Giddens, *The transformation of intimacy* (Cambridge: Polity Press, 1992).

53   De Martino, *La fine del mondo*.

54   Giovanni Jervis, 'Ricordo di Ernesto de Martino. Incontro con Giovanni Jervis', in *Transcultura*, ed. by Antonino Iaria, Maria G. Scalise and Bruno Tagliacozzi (Rome: Edizioni Universitarie Romane, 2000), 35-44 (p. 40).

55   Giovanni Jervis, 'Alcune intuizioni psicologiche di Ernesto de Martino', *Ricerca folklorica*, 13 (1986), 65–67 (p. 66).

56   Jervis, 'Ricordo di Ernesto de Martino', p. 40.

study of tarantism in the Salentine Peninsula,[57] meant viewing the path of possession and ritual dance as first of all a form of psychological support, the redemption from a discomfort that otherwise would spread without structures and contents, thus concealing its aspects of "imprisonment":

> [...] people with neurotic, neurasthenic, or hypochondriac disorders, who underwent that kind of treatment, said they felt good, but after a few months they needed it again [...]; the individuals were taken by a collective mechanism, and hence they ended up being forced to play that role for all their life. So with a twofold regression. From an individual psychological point of view, it was an imprisonment in a mechanism of catharsis without any consciousness raising (because it was indeed a catharsis, but certainly not a catharsis based on insight). From a collective point of view, it was an imprisonment of the whole village; for in being involved in that rite, the community opted for a model of rationalization that was homogeneous to all a series of structures both of thought and social, which had a pre-modern, and indeed feudal character. In that tradition was something essentially immobile, and hence basically conservative.[58]

These final remarks should lead us to disavow the rigid opposition between social (premodern) and individual (late-modern) strategies of coping with crisis. Further inquiry should pursue a critical synthesis of social coping mechanisms and individual emancipation. In other words, while bearing in mind the pathological effects of the 'privatization' of the experience of crisis, theory must also be aware of the risks of regression linked to the one-sided 'socialization' of it. Therefore, we should search for social strategies of protection and restoration of 'presence' which do not foster the organicist integration of individuals within the social whole, but that support psychic integration and a wider emancipation of individuals.

---

57   Ernesto De Martino, *The Land of Remorse*, transl. by Dorothy L. Zinn (London: Free Association Books, 2005).
58   Jervis, 'Ricordo di Ernesto de Martino', pp. 40-41.

MARCO PIAZZA

THE INTERRUPTION OF HABITS AND ITS CONSEQUENCES
Philosophy's Tools and Answers

> It is catastrophe, accident, reaction which brings habit into
> an active condition and creates a habit of changing habits.
> Charles S. Peirce, *New Elements of Mathematics*

1. *Habits, patterns of action, social mimicry*

William James called us a "walking bundle of habits",[1] and John Dewey wrote that man is a "creature of habit",[2] an expression recently revived both by the American philosopher of the mind Alva Noë and by myself.[3] The idea is that our actions are largely attributable to habits learned throughout our existence. A long philosophical tradition rooted in Aristotle considers habits as "permanently acquired dispositions", "inclinations" or "tendencies",[4] which, in a felicitous expression used by Thomas Reid in 1788, take the form of "principles of action".[5] Reid distinguishes between principles of action and "habits of art".[6] The latter are actually what we call

1   William James, 'The Laws of Habit', *Popular Science Monthly*, 30 (1887), 433–51 (pp. 450-51); Id., *Principles of Psychology*, 2 vols (New York: Holt, 1890), I, p. 127.

2   John Dewey, *Human Nature and Conduct. An Introduction to Social Psychology* (New York: Henry Holt and Company, 1922), p. 125.

3   Alva Noë, *Out of Our Heads: Why You Are Not Your Brain, and Other Lessons from the Biology of Consciousness* (New York: Hill and Wang, 2009), p. 97; Marco Piazza, *Creature dell'abitudine. Abito, costume, seconda natura da Aristotele alle scienze cognitive* (Bologna: Il Mulino, 2018), p. 227.

4   See: Thornton C. Lockwood, 'Habituation, Habit and Character in Aristotle's "Nicomachean Ethics"', in Tom Sparrow and Adam Hutchenson (eds.), *A History of Habit. From Aristotle to Bourdieu* (Lanham: Lexington Books, 2013), 19–36.

5   Thomas Reid, 'Essay III Of the Principles of Action', in Id., *Essays on the Active Powers of Man* (1788), ed. by Knud Haakonssen and James A. Harris (Edimburgh: Edimburgh University Press, 2010), 74–195 (p. 88).

6   *Ibid.*

skills or abilities: "if I have acquired a habit of doing something, I have a disposition to do that thing; I am willing to do it. And to be disposed in this sense seems to be more than merely having an ability to do something".[7] Habits are therefore not confined to the routines of our daily lives, but they underpin the complex texture of our behaviour and thoughts. Paraphrasing Bergson, Gilles Deleuze, in his commentary on Hume, proposed to conceive of humans as beings who have "the habit to take up habits".[8] In other words, habit functions as an explanatory principle of our actions and judgements.

If in principle a distinction can be made between individual and social habits — or between private habits and collective customs — it is also true that the former are conditioned by the social context and vice versa. If one of the first things I usually do when I get up is sip a hot cup of coffee, how much has this habit arisen in me independent of the models around me? If I always automatically and unreflectively tie my left shoe before my right, how much does this not depend on the order in which my mother tied my shoes as a child? Of course, I can get used to going without a scarf during the winter, and this depends on my perception of the temperature or my dislike of the garment, but how can I be sure that I have acquired this habit without some form of interaction with the social and cultural models with which I am in contact? In other words, habits are built in a constant dialogue between the individual and the context, and the latter is a natural and cultural, historical and social environment.

In philosophical terms, as Maine de Biran had already guessed, custom is epistemically resolved in habit: it is enough to understand how the latter works to grasp the nature of the former.[9] Moreover, before him, Hume used the emblematic expression "habit or custom", which denotes an almost interchangeable use of the two terms.[10] In the twentieth century, the sociologist who most insisted on the function of habit in explaining our

---

7   Mark Sinclair, 'Habit as Disposition', *Paradigmi*, 38(1), (2020), 9–22 (p. 10).
8   Gilles Deleuze, *Empiricism and Subjectivity. An Essay on Hume's Theory of Human Nature*, trans. by Constantin V. Boundas (New York: Columbia University Press, 1991), p. 44.
9   Maine de Biran, *Influence de l'habitude sur la faculté de penser* (1802), in Id., *Oeuvres, Tome II, Mémoires sur l'habitude*, ed. by Gilbert Romeyer-Dherbey (Paris: Vrin, 1987), 125–90 (p. 160, footnote). The footnote to which I refer is not translated in the English edition by Marguerite D. Boehm, *The Influence of Habit on the Faculty of Thinking* (Baltimore: William and Wilkins, 1929; Westport: Greenwood Press, 1970).
10   John C. Laursen, *The Politics of Skepticism in the Ancients: Montaigne, Hume, and Kant* (Leiden: E.J. Brill, 1992), p. 146.

behaviour and the construction of social ties, namely Pierre Bourdieu, used the Latin term *habitus* to indicate a constellation of phenomena that one of his favourite authors, Pascal, defined, in the wake of Montaigne, as *coutume*, or "custom".[11]

Habit is thus about the formation of patterns of action or patterns of response, produced by our experience but also capable of adapting to the challenges posed by the environment. Thus, our courses of action, i.e. the ways we actually act, depend on patterns that operate as inclinations or tendencies with respect to the choices we make when we decide to act in a certain way. From this point of view, habits are internal instances that arise on the basis of repeated and internalised actions and that are ready to act in new situations, similar to those already experienced.[12]

Patterns of action are like scripts – they are part of the social 'games' we play, and we learn them mainly through imitation: "the appropriation of the world takes place through mimetic activity".[13] In some way we replicate the behaviour of others; we are led to do so by our own brain structure, as neuroscientists now explain through the function of mirror neurons. But with respect to those patterns, those scripts, we are not only receptive, but also active: we can adapt or even transform them.[14] This is precisely because of the brain plasticity that neurology has long postulated, and that current neuroscience defines in terms of a system of neural networks interconnected by synapses that allow the passage of neurotransmitters. This is a dynamic system, in continuous dialogue between inside and outside, which among other things makes the existence of two identical brains impossible.[15]

Our habits therefore represent a battery of action's conducts available as if they were kept in a repository of 'clothes' at hand, i.e. they are

---

11   See: Nick Crossley, 'Pierre Bourdieu's "Habitus"', in Sparrow and Hutchenson, 291–307.

12   See: Beate Kreis, Günter Gebauer, *Habitus* (Bielefeld: Transcript Verlag, 2002), p. 30.

13   Günter Gebauer, 'Praktischer Sinn und Sprache', in Catherine Colliot-Thélène, Étienne François, Günter Gebauer (eds.), *Pierre Bourdieu, Deutsch-französische Perspektiven* (Frankfurt am Main: Suhrkamp, 2005), 137–64 (p. 152).

14   See: Italo Testa, Fausto Caruana, 'The Pragmatist Reappraisal of Habit in Contemporary Cognitive Science, Neuroscience, and Social Theory: Introductory Essay', in Fausto Caruana, Italo Testa (eds.), *Habits. Pragmatist Approaches from Cognitive Science, Neuroscience, and Social Theory* (Cambridge, Cambridge University Press, 2021), 1–37.

15   See: Catherine Malabou, *What Should We Do with Our Brain?* trans by Sebastian Rand (New York: Fordham University Press, 2008).

ready responses, activated in certain circumstances without apparent reflexive mediation. This does not mean that they do not contain a trace of intentionality (which in some cases causes them, but not always).[16] The hunter who, sensing the swoosh of a bird behind him, turns and shoots without thinking and apparently without even aiming, has to some extent decided to go along with that sequence of gestures that have become automatic for him. That is, he could have, for some reason, exercised his attention to block that sequence or to modify it according to an evaluation of contingent factors.[17] Similarly, a gesture repeated hundreds of times in an almost identical manner within some collective ritual, religious or secular, may be performed differently based on a reconsideration of the context or meaning of that gesture.

Our habits are thus the effect of processes of interaction with the environment in which we absorb patterns of action and behaviours that correspond to cultural sedimentation, sometimes of long duration, but on closer inspection are always also susceptible to modification and revision. Philosophers have often reserved for themselves the role of innovators, insisting on the emancipatory function of philosophy in relation to our habits, understood as social practices reflecting worldviews, prejudices, superstitions, and fanaticisms. They also developed theorisations capable of accounting for our imitative nature without locking us into a determinism that would make us passive automatons enslaved to our instincts like animals. One of them dates to 1755 and is contained in the *Treatise of Animals*, in which Condillac establishes a comparison between man and animals on the question of instinct and imitation. First of all, he starts from the recognition of habits as abilities: "habits arise from the need to exercise one's faculties: hence the number of habits is proportionate to the number of needs". But "beasts evidently have fewer needs than we do", and "as soon as they know how to feed themselves, how to shelter themselves from the ravages of the wind, how to defend themselves from their enemies, and how to flee from them, they know all that is necessary for their preservation". The animals thus contract the same habits, and this happens among them in the same way as it would "if they lived separately, without any kind of relationship, and therefore without being able to imitate each other". This is because between them, according to Condillac,

---

16   See: Bill Pollard, 'Identification, Psychology, and Habits', in Jesús Aguilar, Andrei A. Buckareff, Keith Frankish (eds.), *New Waves in Philosophy of Action* (Basingstoke: Palgrave Macmillan, 2010), 81–97.

17   See: Christos Douskos, 'Deliberation and Automaticity in Habitual Acts', *Ethics in Progress*, 9, 2018(1), 25–43.

"there is very little exchange", even at an intraspecific level. Thus, animals "begin the same studies again at each generation", unlike humans, who "communicate needs, experiences, imitate each other", giving rise to "a mass of knowledge that grows from one generation to the next". Moreover, the needs that humans communicate to each other are not those that are "absolutely necessary for conservation", in respect to which they act exactly in the same way as animals, responding with "operations, which are the same in each of them, [...] for which they do not think of imitating themselves at all". These are more complex needs, which are added to the fundamental ones as the structure of society becomes more articulated and culture is modified, thanks precisely to human nature, which is imitative and creates potentially infinite combinations. Each human being "does not merely imitate one man, he imitates all those who approach him, so he resembles no one exactly". However, with respect to the progress that human knowledge achieves, there are few individuals who really promote it: the majority are "slavish imitators", while "extremely rare" are the "inventors", i.e. those who add something substantial to what they find already established or help to modify it.[18]

2. Changes in habits and the tendency to restore balance

Between the end of the nineteenth and the beginning of the twentieth century, Émile Durkheim developed a theory that to some extent represents an ideal continuation of Condillac's. At first he clarified that habit acts both in simple societies — where "the most puerile customs become categorical duties from force of habit"[19] and where habit "exerts over both people and things a sway that lacks any countervailing force", given "living conditions almost invariably"[20] — and in complex ones, based on the division of labour, in which the "organisation necessarily implies an absolute regularity in habits, for a change cannot occur in the mode of functioning of an organ without its having repercussions upon the whole organism".[21] Regarding the latter, however, in accordance with the classic idea of the force of habit that (for better or worse) opposes resistance to change, he only reiterates

---

18 Étienne Bonnot de Condillac, *Traité des animaux*, in Id., *Oeuvres philosophiques*, ed. by Georges Le Roy, 3 vols (Paris: PUF, 1947-1951), I, 339–79 (pp. 358b-360a).
19 Émile Durkheim, *The Division of Labour in Society*, trans. by Wilfred D. Halls (Houndmills & London: Macmillan, 1984), p. 111.
20 *Ibid.*, p. LIII.
21 *Ibid.*, p. 187.

that the change of mentality occurs slowly because "it is always a laborious operation to uproot habits that time has fixed and organised within us".[22] Sometime later, based on the reading of American pragmatists, in particular Peirce and Dewey, he returned to his theory, specifying that "when balance is disturbed in a living organism, consciousness awakes", and then fades "when it no longer serves a purpose. It only awakes when habit is disrupted, when a process on non-adaption occurs".[23] In other words, the possibility of change occurs when our behavioural automatisms, which are largely social automatisms, are interrupted by some resistance they encounter in their actualization.

Changes in habits can therefore occur abruptly. It happens when an unexpected event blocks an association made stable by habit, as in a famous example contained in Descartes' *Passions of the Soul*, aimed at showing that it is possible to interrupt one associative scheme and replace it with another. To this end, even a single action may be necessary, as when, so to speak involuntarily,

> we unexpectedly come upon something very foul in a dish we are eating with relish and the surprise that is thus determined may so change the disposition of our brain that we cannot afterwards look upon any such food without repulsion, whereas previously we ate it with pleasure.[24]

According to others, such as Léon Dumont, for many habits, individual and collective, things are not so simple. The organs of our bodies have limits in terms of changes in structure and size: an athlete, for example, cannot acquire greater muscle strength beyond a certain stage. In other words, our physiology is the result of very long processes of adaptation to the environment, so that "individual changes are limited mainly by hereditary and congenital structure".[25] But even when a change is made possible by the elasticity of our psychophysical structures, the power of established habits is such that they can regain the upper hand over newly acquired habits: "the habits of recent date, which have succeeded in triumphing momentarily over old habits, are soon cancelled out by the latter, unless

---

22 Durkheim, p. 186.
23 Émile Durkheim, *Pragmatism and Sociology*, ed. by John B. Allcock, trans. by John C. Whitehouse (Cambridge: Cambridge University Press, 1983), p. 79.
24 René Descartes, *The Passions of the Soul*, trans. by John Cottingham, Robert Stoohoff, and Dugald Murdoch, in Id., *The Philosophical Writings*, 3 vols (Cambridge, Cambridge University Press, 1985), I, 325–404 (p. 348).
25 Léon Dumont, 'L'Habitude', *Revue philosophique de la France et de l'Étranger*, 1, 1876(1), 321–66 (p. 363).

they are kept active by frequent repetition".[26] In other words, according to Dumont, "the new habit is continually threatened, attacked by the return of its adversary; and, unless it finds succour in the renewal of excitement from without, it resists less and less".[27] A clear example given by Dumont is political. A revolution, triggered by a few, finds the consent of the many because of the negative living conditions a regime has imposed upon them, and in this way a new political and social order very quickly replaces the previous one, which may have lasted for decades if not centuries. But the force of habit is such that the old order presses on, and revolutions are often followed by restorations. This is also because "an overthrown government leaves behind it interests and habits which work continually for it, ready to take advantage, to regain ground, of the inevitable mistakes of the new government, which always encounters, because of its novelty, immense difficulties of adaptation".[28] If we correspond to systems of habits, as Dumont proposes us to consider, we are therefore the actors in a struggle between habits which takes place both at an individual and at a social level: "established habits resist the introduction of new habits; and old habits react for a long time against relatively recently acquired habits".[29] It must be concluded, as Dumont writes, that "the greatest enemy of habit is habit itself"![30]

Dumont is not only one of the very few philosophers of habit to have dwelt on the dynamics of the interruption of one habit and its sudden replacement by another, but he has also shown how the process of adaptation within which individuals and human societies develop their complex systems of habits — "systems of systems", in his terminology — is not necessarily a positive one: "not all adaptations are equally happy and fruitful achievements. The vices of the individual and the bad habits of peoples are themselves habits, so that alongside the seeds of progress there may also be causes of decline".[31] In other words, just as human beings can become accustomed to vices or self-destructive behaviour, societies can also take the path of decline, which in a sense is the equivalent for human groups of the risk of extinction for animal species. And if there is an antidote to this process of involution, humans find it difficult to identify it:

---

26 Dumont, p. 364.
27 *Ibid.*
28 *Ibid.*
29 *Ibid.*
30 Dumont, p. 363.
31 Dumont, p. 365.

a habit that has assumed an excessive and disproportionate development has unfortunately a greater chance than others of being further increased and strengthened, because it imposes itself in an exclusive manner, generates more imperious needs and is, consequently, exercised more often; while the weaker and more tenuous habits, which it would be necessary to exercise to a greater extent to re-establish equilibrium, are usually those that one is more willing to neglect. It is thus very difficult to get out of a bad road when one has entered it the first time.[32]

Once again, we find the reference to the power of habit and its intrinsic ambivalence. And Dumont's explanation of the dynamics of social decline is quite convincing, since "public opinion cannot be against the habits of the majority; it can only blame what is accidental, exceptional, more or less rare".[33] In this way, it does not realise that the cause of its decline is right in front of it, in its own customs: evil is to be found "where, as a consequence, it is less likely to be sought, and where the force of tradition and opinion, that is to say, of custom, would probably make any change difficult".[34]

Dumont's examples and the theories recalled so far help us to define an epistemic framework within which to situate our recent experience, namely the sudden interruption of our habits because of an unexpected event reasonably experienced as catastrophic, namely the pandemic. Before addressing the analysis of current events, however, it may be useful to recall another of the rare theories that has considered the consequences of the interruption of a habit: the philosophy of habit contained in Marcel Proust's *In Search of Lost Time*. Here, it is very clear that without habit, our life would be constantly exposed to the anguish of the unknown: thanks to habit, albeit progressively, a living space, an environment, is made habitable:

> Habit! The skilful but slow-moving arranger who begins by letting our minds suffer for weeks on end in temporary quarters, but whom our minds are none the less only too happy to discover at last, for without it, reduced to their own devices, they would be powerless to make any room seem habitable.[35]

---

32   *Ibid.*
33   *Ibid.*
34   Dumont, p. 366.
35   Marcel Proust, *In Search of Lost Time*, trans. by Charles K. Scott Moncrieff and Terence Kilmartin, revised by Dennis J. Enright, 6 vols (New York: The Modern Library, 1992-1993), I, 8–9.

Proust invokes the habituating power of habit as a beneficial element that puts an end to the hypersensitivity of our soul and reconciles us with the context in which we find ourselves. The system of our habits acts in the same way as a drug that takes a certain amount of time for its beneficial effects to be felt, and more precisely as the kind of drug that does not treat the causes of illness but its symptoms, so that discontinuing it can make them reappear immediately. Hence the need for what is habitual, well exemplified by the need of the protagonist of the novel, when he is a child, to receive a goodnight kiss from his mother before falling asleep, which, like a medicine to which one slowly becomes accustomed, generates an additional need, that of a second kiss before the mother leaves her son's room:

> the concession which she made to my wretchedness and agitation in coming up to give me this kiss of peace always annoyed my father, who thought such rituals absurd, and she would have liked to try to induce me to outgrow the need, the habit, of having her there at all, let alone get into the habit of asking her for an additional kiss when she was already crossing the threshold.[36]

The interruption of a habit thus proves to be a very painful event. The novel's protagonist experiences this quite harshly once he has become a young man, in the development of his love affair with Albertine, the girl towards whom he feels a passion deeply imbued with jealousy. When he realises that his beloved feels only affection for him and that he is therefore in danger of being abandoned by her, he simulates a separation to provoke a rapprochement, but he does not realise that by doing so he deprives himself of "the solid ground of habit upon which to rest, even in one's sorrow".[37] It is a game in which one pretends to be able to get along without the other while having as a result the exact opposite effect, a game that makes us "suffer anew because one has created something new and unfamiliar which thus resembles those cures that are destined in time to heal the malady from which one is suffering, but the first effects of which are to aggravate it".[38] That evil is none other than amorous passion, against whose paralysing routine the protagonist implements cures that fail, bringing out the painful core of the relationship, anchored to habits, as well as the very poverty of passion, not nourished by the partner who is the object of the protagonist's exasperating possessiveness. It is precisely the disappearance

---

36   Proust, I, 15.
37   Proust, V, 477.
38   Proust, V, 477-78.

of the beloved that brings out the full extent of the possibility, intrinsically inherent in habit, of producing pain. This latter aspect often goes unnoticed, hidden as it is by the positive one, that is, by its soothing, anaesthetising character, by its "annihilating force, which suppresses the originality and even the awareness of one's perceptions",[39] as Proust points out, in perfect harmony with much previous philosophy, from Hume to Maine de Biran and Ravaisson.

With the sudden disappearance of Albertine, the veil of habit is suddenly torn and this is revealed in one of its two faces, the negative one that makes it

> a dread deity, so riveted to one's being, its insignificant face so incrusted in one's heart, that if it detaches itself, if it turns away from one, this deity that one had barely distinguished inflicts upon on one sufferings more terrible than any other and is then as cruel as death itself.[40]

However, this is not the only perspective provided by Proust's *In Search of Lost Time* on the relationship between habit and the sphere of pleasure and pain. The breaking away from habits can also produce pleasure, not only pain: "when I found myself turn from my habits — in a new place, or going out at an unaccustomed hour — I was feeling a lively pleasure".[41] So, when the interruption is voluntary and deliberate, guided by a curious and experimental intentionality, the suspension of the habit does not involve painful consequences, but rather proves to be a generator of new experiences and therefore a potential source of pleasure.[42] In other words, it is a guided and supervised process, active and not passive, in which the mental aspect prevails over the passionate one.

3. *Habits and pandemic*

Moving on to current events, let us try to apply to the disorientating experience of the pandemic the interpretative coordinates that have guided the millennial reflection of Western philosophies of habit. First of all, we are faced with unforeseen risks, with effects not only on individuals, but on entire communities, indeed on the world population. There is therefore a global

---

39   Proust, V, 564.
40   Proust, V, 564-65.
41   Proust, VI, 253.
42   Piazza, p. 165.

dimension, and equally, a global fear. The pandemic, in addition to its health and indirect socio-economic effects, is not only a pandemic of the virus, but also a pandemic of fear. The measures applied to contain the pandemic, combined with the fear generated by the spread of the virus, i.e. by the pandemic itself, has led to a sudden interruption of almost all of our lifestyles, which can be seen in exemplary fashion through the prism of lockdown periods.

During the different phases of confinement, but also during the intermediate and subsequent phases of less rigid restrictions applied over the months that followed in an alternating pattern, it was not only habits related to social interaction and movement that were suspended. The rhythms of life and our relationship with home environments have been subverted, and the rarefied nature of human exchanges has severely affected our perception of reality and the quality of our psychophysical balance. Since we were not prepared, we experienced this situation as a traumatic event, and felt the pain of the sudden interruption of our needs, rituals, and ways of life.

There is a whole series of habits that could not be replaced with others that were similar or suited to filling certain needs. The use of the mask and social distancing did not produce better experiences of relationships than those known until then. The forms of sensory interaction, related to touch and smell, not to mention sexual ones, did not find an equivalent in video calls on Skype or other similar platforms, where the only sensory channels were sight and hearing.

In other cases, the suspension of certain habits coincided with their replacement by others – a substitution that was forced, induced, and therefore painful because it was not desired. In some cases, however, it proved to be productive of new experiences, which filled the void left by the interrupted and suspended habits. Confinement within the home and forced cohabitation among family members did not necessarily lead to a worsening of social ties or to an escalation of domestic violence. Or rather, this happened when the individuals involved in such situations did not take advantage of the new situation to try to activate themselves, producing alternative forms of life, resilient responses to the new state of things. Thus, a first piece of evidence concerns the value that in similar circumstances assumes the capacity to be active subjects who practice the elaboration of new habits to replace previous ones, in this case interrupted due to an external cause. For this to be possible, it is necessary to be aware of our plasticity, of the potential we have to modify our habits and adapt them to the changing context, even when it is rapid and catches us unawares.

However, the experience of the pandemic also showed us another aspect of the dynamics of habits: that whereby old, established habits struggle to get the better of newly introduced habits. We witnessed an initial phase of positive adaptation, in which we implemented response strategies based on solidarity and the maintenance of communication and relationships, albeit at a distance and in new forms. We thus tried to acquire new relational habits, together with a series of new hygienic-sanitary habits: in addition to the use of masks, continuous hygienisation, with unprecedented attention to the cleaning of spaces, surfaces and environments, etc. But as the perception of risk has diminished, either because of the progress of mass vaccination or because of a psychological mechanism of habituation, we have begun to resume many old habits. And if, in some cases, the situation has forced us to readjust our old ones to the new context, our expectation is to be able to return as soon as possible to our previous practices, to our old way of life.

All this shows that we are eager to restore old habits, without being able to make a broader assessment of their intrinsic value. If the pandemic can also be seen as an effect of the wrong relationship between man and the environment, i.e. if it is one of the many faces of a dangerous and careless exploitation of the ecosystem in which we live, we should carefully consider which habits to restore and which not to restore, which to modify and which to correct. Otherwise, we could risk slipping further down that sloping plane that has thrown us into the present condition and which seems to correspond more to a phase of decline than to one of progress in the history of the evolution of the human species.[43] In other words, it is a question of placing the pandemic within a broader context that assesses our relationship with the environment, thus considering it not only as a health emergency, but as one of the alarm bells sounded by the ecosystem in which we live, with respect to which we continue to behave inconsiderately.[44] This is a situation that requires a change of perspective with regard to our self-perception in relation to the universe, i.e. our place in the universe.

However, the experience of the pandemic has also confronted us with a significant potential that we tend to underestimate in the more routine phases of our existence, both as individuals and as members of our

---

43   See: Claire Colebrook, *Death of the PostHuman. Essays on Extinction. Vol. 1* (London: Open Humanities Press, 2014), pp. 29–44.
44   See: Thomas S. Cowan, Sally Fallon Morell, *The Contagyon Myth. Why Viruses (including "Coronavirus") Are Not the Cause of Disease* (New York: Skyhorse Publishing, 2020).

collective entities. In other words, it made us experience first-hand our flexibility and adaptability. In a very short period, we have been able to restructure our daily life, our rituals, and our habitual behaviours, sacrificing very important portions of our relational and social spheres and trying to compensate for 'losses' with 'gains' that were unthinkable until recently. It is then a question of directing our capacities in a constructive direction and not just a defensive one. That is, we can train ourselves to respond to other similar future risk situations.[45] And this will already be an advantage: if the state of risk should persist, we will be able to develop a level of attention capable of making us change habits rapidly, as if we had different clothes at our disposal, different patterns, interchangeable as it were.

Someone recently spoke of "elastic habits", referring to the individual sphere.[46] This concept can be extended to the social sphere, especially since there is no separation between inside and outside when we refer to habits: they are patterns of action elaborated from outside and modified by both internal and external inputs. In other words, we internalise the social world outside, but we also have the power to change it in the process of individualization.[47]

However, our elasticity in terms of habits, to which our cerebral plasticity corresponds, has limits: there are spheres of our experience that cannot be cancelled or excessively reduced without incalculable or irreversible damage. This is because the consequences of this type of event on our psychophysical balance are deleterious in the long run and our behavioural plasticity cannot compensate for certain deficiencies generated by them beyond a certain limit.

As we know, the pandemic has had negative effects on our socialisation processes, on the quality of our social relationships. Virtual reality and digital media have to some extent mitigated these effects, but certainly a long continuation of the restrictions we experienced with the lockdown could have negative consequences on our mental health, as is already indicated by the increase in mental pathologies (especially depression, acts of violence against oneself, suicidal tendencies, etc.) even among minors,

---

45   See: David Mariani, Raffaele Picco, Francesca Capitanini, Alex Porciani, Marco Lombardi, Luigi Capotondo, Alessandro Capitanini, 'Le abitudini al tempo del Coronavirus', *Giornale di clinica nefrologica e dialisi*, 32 (2020), 69–72.

46   Stephen Guise, *Elastic Habits. How to Create Smarter Habits That Adapt to Your Day* (Windermere: Selective Entertainment LLC, 2019).

47   See: Italo Testa, 'A Habit Ontology for Cognitive and Social Sciences. Methodological Individualism, Pragmatist Interactionism, and 4E Cognition', in Caruana and Testa, pp. 395–416.

and in deviant and aggressive behaviour: intra-family violence, feminicide, etc.[48] In fact, all the multisensory aspects of human interaction have been neutralised by distancing and limitations, greatly reducing the quality of our experience. This is a risk we must try to avoid by building new habits of life, of consumption, of relationship with the environment, capable of reducing the danger of new pandemics and of extreme measures to contain them, such as lockdown. In other words, we must use our flexibility to devise new living scenarios in which the risk of pandemics is contained and reduced.

---

48   See: Maria-Elizabeth Loades, Eleanor Chatburn, Nina Higson-Sweeney, Shirley Reynolds, Roz Shafran, Amberly Brigden, Catherine Linney, Megan Niamh McManus, Catherine Borwick, Esther Crawley, 'Rapid Systematic Review: The Impact of Social Isolation and Loneliness on the Mental Health of Children and Adolescents in the Context of COVID-19', *Journal of the American Academy of Child & Adolescent Psychiatry*, 59, 2020(11), 1218–1239; Livia Tomova, Kimberly L. Wang, Todd Thompson, Gillian A. Matthews, Atsushi Takahashi, Key M. Tye, and Rebecca Saxe, 'Acute social isolation evokes midbrain craving responses similar to hunger', *Natural Neurosciences*, 23 (2020), 1597–1605; Hai-Xin Bo, Wen Li, Yuan Yang, Yu Wang, Qinge Zhang, Teris Cheung, Xinjuan Wu, Yu-Tao Xiang, 'Posttraumatic stress symptoms and attitude toward crisis mental health services among clinically stable patients with COVID-19 in China', *Psychological Medicine*, 51(6) (2021), pp. 1052–1053.

CORINNA GUERRA

A NATURAL RISK WE CAN LIVE WITH[1]
A Tentative Parallel

1. *What viruses and volcanoes have in common*

As historians we are used to dealing with pandemics, but this time it is different: the current pandemic affects us all personally, now. We can thus appreciate how powerful philosophical reasoning could be on our view of habits, those constitutive parts of ourselves and our societies, as we now feel ourselves deprived of them. On the other hand, one who works on volcanoes – perhaps the most mysterious subject of inquiry of the eighteenth century – from an environmental humanities point of view can easily recognize a powerful multidimensional tool to study landscapes, people's behaviors, and societies. It happens that an unexpected and invisible factor erupted into our personal and professional lives in 2019, a new member of the Coronavirus family which began to directly threaten our daily routines. Suddenly, experts of natural risk and those who study habits were walking in the same research field.

In fact, studying volcanic eruptions, above all during a period in which volcanic phenomena were not framed in scientific theory, means to analyze what happens to people's lives before and after the eruption and to understand how the simple presence of the active volcano shapes people's behaviors in the absence of the actual eruptive event.

When the new coronavirus became the disease of 2019, and then a pandemic, our collective and personal habits were affected with some consequences on politics, education, the economy, and so on. This is similar to what we see on the occasion of catastrophic volcanic eruptions. To name

1   This paper is a starting work for the author's research funded by the project FARE *EarlyGeoPraxis* (Grant from the Italian Ministry of University and Research, cod. R184WNSTWH) and it also contributes to the project ERC *EarlyModernCosmology* (Horizon 2020, GA 725883). The author thanks the Max Planck Partner Group *The Water City* (Max Planck Institute for the History of Science, Berlin, in collaboration with Ca' Foscari University of Venice).

just a few examples, there is an impressive phenomenon that occurs during large eruptions, where falling ash obscures the sky. To understand just how shocking this phenomenon could be, it is worth noting that the inhabitants of Sumbawa Island gave a name to the enormous 1815 Tambora volcanic eruption: the Time of the Ash Rain, which also inspired Byron's poem *Darkness*.[2] The global impact of that event was due precisely to the plumes of Tambora ash travelling all over the world for years by means of winds and the great energy of the explosion. This ash, which obscured the sun, caused the "year without summer", and as a consequence, a famine.[3] Very recently, and thus more relevant to the present-day disruption of daily routines, was the eruption of Eyjafjallajökull in Iceland, which led to an unprecedented blockade of air traffic. Today, in fact, regarding the global effects of large volcanic events, the focus of scientists is on how ash can affect air traffic, how to foresee the eruptions, and how to manage them quickly enough.[4]

If we can easily draw some similarities between the explosion of a pandemic and that of a volcano, we cannot forget the important difference that, as stated before, volcanic territory is all the time a natural risk place, even when there are not eruptive events. If an eruption and a pandemic have in common the fact that they explode without warning, immediately disrupting our lives, in the case of a volcanic landscape, people will experience a much less traumatic disruption to their daily lives and habits. This is due to the fact that people living in volcanic territories have likely developed habits that have adapted them to living in the presence of a natural hazard.

Might a virus pandemic become our world's natural risk, one we learn to live with even when there are no pandemics traveling around the world?

---

2   Gillen D'Arcy Wood, *Tambora: the eruption that changed the world* (Princeton, Oxford: Princeton University Press, 2014), pp. 24; 67.
3   Manuel Pineiro Vaquero, 2015. 'Introduzione. Rileggere le carestie di Antico Regime: tra Food Availability Decline e Entitlements', in Maria Luisa Ferrari and Manuel Pineiro Vaquero (ed. by), *Moia la carestia: la scarsità alimentare in età preindustriale* (Bologna: Il Mulino, 2015), 9–22 (p. 11).
4   Roberto Suipizio and others, 'Hazard assessment of far-range volcanic ash dispersal from a violent Strombolian eruption at Somma-Vesuvius volcano, Naples, Italy: implications on civil aviation', *Bulletin of volcanology*, 74(9) (2012), 2205-2218. Of course, the Eyjafjallajökull eruption generated a consistent flow of publications, just to list one work interesting for our aims: Paolo Rossini and others, 'April-May 2010 Eyjafjallajökull Volcanic Fallout over Rimini, Italy', *Atmospheric Environment*, 48 (2012), 122–28 Web.

This is something that came to mind when considering the disruption of habits we experienced in 2020. It is now quite common to use past events in order to improve the perception and prevention of volcanic risk. This is possible because, for example, the current generation has not had direct experience of a volcanic eruption, but they live with the risk of one. As they have the menace of the volcano, they have an understanding of the range of vulnerabilities they live with.[5] Understanding the vulnerabilities means thinking about evacuation capacity, road practicability, hospital capacity, and other parameters that must be related to population density. We similarly learned last year about the vulnerabilities relating to the speed of contagion, for example. In short, risk is the result of a threat, perhaps a danger, plus vulnerability and potential harm (harm should be interpreted in a broad sense, which means to consider physical, structural, and psychological harm). The result of all these estimations is that we can live in a territory of risk by means of the habits we inherited from our ancestors. How much people are conscious of that is still an object of debate, since risk perception is not something that can be quantified, as we all have experienced in the past months.

One of the characteristics of the study of earthquakes, as well as volcanic eruptions, is that the historian should account for very different practices and knowledge systems.[6] From archival research to geology and chemistry, it is a transdisciplinary job, difficult to place within narrow epistemological limits.[7] A too narrow approach by the social sciences could hide the dichotomy between the man monopole on the transformation of nature and the work of nature itself, which has no intentionality, but a materiality that we are forced to take into account. This is the main characteristic of volcanoes as natural risk – people living in these territories are not allowed to ignore the presence of risk in their daily routines. The price of ignoring it in daily individual and social practices is to suffer a more severe trauma than expected when the natural risk event occurs. This is a facet of the complex and rich relationship

---

5   Jelle Zeilinga De Boer and Donald Theodore Sanders, *Volcanoes in Human History: The Far-Reaching Effects of Major Eruptions* (Princeton, Oxford: Princeton University Press, 2002), p. xii.

6   Anne Marie Granet-Abisset, 'L'historien, les risques et l'environnement : un regard sur la nature et les hommes', David Thevenot, *23èmes Journées Scientifiques de l'Environnement - Risques environnementaux: détecter, comprendre, s'adapter*, January 31st – February 2nd, 2012 at the Hôtel du Département à Créteil, Créteil, France, 10 (2013).

7   Giacomo Parrinello, *Fault lines: earthquakes and urbanism in modern Italy* (New York, Oxford: Berghahn, 2015), p. 4.

between humans and their environment. Natural landscapes are not only a physical space where people can move, but an active part of their lives. Natural disasters or pandemics come to remind us how important and peculiar this relationship is.

In the case of volcanoes, a crucial moment to test this opposition might be the end of the eighteenth century. Moreover it is the power of a virus, which is just a small agglomeration of genetic information and of the proteins encoded therein, that caused the health crisis we have suffered over the last two years. One thing they have clearly in common: the volcanic event and the pandemic are processes perfectly inscribed between a before and an after, an integral part of society[8] and of its biophysical environment. From this point of view, they must be considered on the opposite side of an isolated, unforeseeable event as sometimes it is interpreted.

The reactions of people and of institutions, and the development of new knowledge and practices, shows the influence the presence of the volcano has on the population living nearby and of the virus pandemic on global humanity.[9] It might be useful, then, to build upon the concept of risk and the antecedent one of menace.[10] The tools of the historian studying the prediction and prevention of natural risks, which are in general linked with the territory,[11] now could be applied to a risk deprived of its territorial origin.

---

8   Christof Mauch and Christian Pfister (ed. by), *Natural Disasters, Cultural Responses: Case Studies toward a Global Environmental History*, (Lanham, Boulder, New York, Toronto, and Plymouth, UK: Lexington Books, 2009). Adelina Miranda, 'The temporal polysemy of risk: when the words of men of science meet the interpretations of the inhabitants in the Vesuvius Region', *Temporalités*, 1 (2004), 5-21, online 23 June 23, 2009 (last access: November 14th, 2021).

9   "L'idée de nature contient une quantité extraordinaire d'histoire humaine, la réciproque est vraie". Gregory Quenet, *Versailles, une histoire naturelle* (Paris: La Découverte, 2015), quoting Raymond Williams, p. 9.

10   François Walter, Bernardino Fantini, Pascal Delvaux (ed. by), *Les cultures du risque* (XVIe-XXIe s.), (Geneva: Presses d'Histoire Suisse, 2006), p. X. Rosmarie Zeller, 'Les catastrophes naturelles au début de l'époque moderne. Entre curiosité, événement terrifiant et interprétation religieuse', Réné Favier and Anne Marie Granet-Abisset (ed. by), *Récits et représentations des catastrophes depuis l'Antiquité* (Grenoble: CNRS-MSH-Alpes, 2004); François Walter, 'Pour une histoire culturelle des risques naturels', Walter, Fantini, Delvaux (ed. by), paragraph 1.

11   Anne Marie Granet-Abisset and Stéphane Gal (ed. by), *Les territoires du risque. Villes, environnement, territoires: Regards croisés sur l'environnement* (Grenoble:

2. Habits for pandemics as a natural risk

The importance of epidemics on the development of human society can hardly be underestimated.[12] Yet their social and economic relevance is expected to rise due to a combination of the long-range mobility of humans and the population increase. The density and size of human agglomeration is increasing,[13] and the probability that humans and their domesticated animals will get in contact with wild organisms affected by zoonosis is enhanced by the exploitation of the natural environment with dramatic reductions in natural ecosystems and biodiversity. The number of people attending to domestic animals has increased exponentially, and never before has there been so much opportunity for pathogens to pass from wild and domestic animals to affect people causing zoonoses. The result has been a worldwide increase in epidemic outbreaks and the persistence of neglected zoonotic diseases in poor countries.[14] A recent study based on epidemics from 1600 to contemporary times estimated that experiencing a COVID-19-like pandemic in one's lifetime is now up to 38%, with the likelihood of doubling in the near future.[15]

Thus, COVID-19 will be not only the pandemic of 2019-2022, but the first of a series of many virus pandemics.[16] We must look to our ancestors' habits during past pandemics for guidance.

Presses Universitaires de Grenoble, 2015), *Avant-propos*; Émilie-Anne Pépy, 'Montagne(s) des naturalistes: l'invention de territoires scientifiques, XVIe-XIXe siècle', Anne Marie Granet-Abisset and Stéphane Gal (ed. by), pp. 163–78. Adelina Miranda, 'Les multiples représentations du risque dans la région de Naples', Walter, Fantini, Delvaux (ed. by), p. 155.

12 Jo N. Hays, *Epidemics and pandemics: their impacts on human history* (Santa Barbara, Calif.: ABC-CLIO, 2005).

13 Max Roser, Hannah Ritchie and Esteban Ortiz-Ospina, 'World Population Growth' (Published online at OurWorldInData.org). <https://ourworldindata.org/world-population-growth> (last access: November 17th, 2021).

14 Delia Grace and others, 'Zoonoses: Blurred lines of emergent disease and ecosystem health', UNEP, *UNEP Frontiers 2016 Report: Emerging issues of environmental concern* (Nairobi, Kenya: United Nations Environment Programme, 2016), 18-30.

15 Marco Marani and others, 'Intensity and frequency of extreme novel epidemics', *Proceedings of the National Academy of Sciences*, 118, 2021(35), e2105482118.

16 David Quammen, *Spillover: animal infections and the next human pandemic* (New York: W. W. Norton & Company, 2012). "Since 2009, the US Agency for International Development has supported the PREDICT project in 35 countries and US research institutions to provide proof of concept that collecting samples from host species can lead to important scientific findings. The Prince Mahidol Awards Conference in 2018 in Bangkok, Thailand, highlighted the importance of the topic: 'Global trends indicate that new microbial threats will continue to

At this point, our historical analysis meets some uncertainty: in fact, after every epidemic of the twenty-first century, we knew more about the viruses, but forgot all about the events themselves. That is unfortunate, since what happened to people's habits during and after a pandemic gives us the opportunity to quantify risk and then to learn how to live with risk.

> We didn't have the time to take out the dead. We left them stacked in a room beneath the urgent care ward. And we took them out when we could, during the day or evening. People arrived on stretchers in terrible shape. They were dying of pulmonary hemorrhage, their lips cyanotic, all gray. There were of all ages, 20, 30, 40 and over. That lasted 10 to 15 days and then it calmed down. And strangely, we have forgotten.[17]

These words were pronounced by a resuscitation physician who worked in a French hospital during the winter of 1969-1970. These words sound too close to ones we have become accustomed to, yet the physician was referring to the so-called 1968 Hong Kong flu, responsible for 20,000 deaths in Italy in just a matter of weeks.[18]

---

emerge at an accelerating rate, driven by our growing population, expanded travel and trade networks, and human encroachment into wildlife habitat. Most emerging viruses are zoonotic, that is, transferred between vertebrates and humans'". Quotations from Olga Jonas and Richard Seifman, 'Do we need a Global Virome Project?', *The Lancet. Global health*, vol. 7(10) (2019), e1314-e1316 (last access: November 11th, 2021). See also Helene Branswell, 'Finding the world's unknown viruses–before they find us', December 13th, 2016 <https://www.statnews.com/2016/12/13/world-viruses-global-virome-project/> (last access: November 15th, 2021); Dennis Carroll and others, 'The Global Virome Project', *Science* (New York, N.Y.), vol. 359,6378 (2018), 872-74. The Global Virome Project official website <https://www.globalviromeproject.org/>. Please, pay your attention to the fact that are all studies published before the actual SARS-CoV-2 pandemic.

17 "On n'avait pas le temps de sortir les morts. On les entassait dans une salle au fond du service de réanimation. Et on les évacuait quand on pouvait, dans la journée, le soir. Les gens arrivaient en brancard, dans un état catastrophique. Ils mouraient d'hémorragie pulmonaire, les lèvres cyanosées, tout gris. Il y en avait de tous les âges, 20, 30, 40 ans et plus.
Ça a duré dix à quinze jours, et puis ça s'est calmé. Et étrangement, on a oublié". Pr. Pierre Dellamonica, that time resuscitation physician at the hospital Edouard-Herriot of Lyon, Winter 1969-70. Corinne Bensimon, *Libération*, 17 December 2005, quoted by Arnaud Fontanet, Episode 2: Impact des pandémies et nouvelles réponses face aux émergences infectieuses, Série Épidémiologie, problématiques et enjeux (8 episodes), Les Cours du Collège de France, February 2019.

18 *Le Pandemie Influenzali del Ventesimo Secolo1968: Influenza Hong Kong (H3N2)* <https://www.epicentro.iss.it/passi/storiePandemia (last access: November 15th,

Why did we so quickly and totally erase the memory of another virus pandemic in recent history? The warning signs were all at our disposal, as well as our good intentions.[19] Yet another example is the SARS (Severe Acute Respiratory Syndrome) epidemic of 2002-2003,[20] or the frightening Ebola virus epidemic (EDV) of 2013-2016. It was a piece of news a few days ago of this writing that the Prix Galien Italy 2021 was awarded to the vaccine against Ebola Msd,[21] yet Ebola cases are still being diagnosed.[22] EVD was declared a public health emergency of international concern by the director of the World Health Organization on August 8th, 2014 and an emergency state was activated until March 29th of 2016.[23] It seemed clear to everyone that we were experiencing the new age of recurring epidemics, as

---

2021). Bojan Pancevski, 'Forgotten Pandemic Offers Contrast to Today's Coronavirus Lockdowns; In the late 1960s, the Hong Kong Flu was allowed to run rampant until a vaccine was introduced', *The Wall Street Journal. Eastern Edition*, 24 April 2020 Web.

19   'SARS is a warning,' Gro Harlem Brundtland, Former Director-General of the World Health Organization, explained. "SARS pushed even the most advanced public health systems to a tipping point. These protections have held, but only barely. Next time, we may not be so lucky. We have an opportunity now, and we see clearly what we need, to rebuild public health defences. They will be needed for the next global epidemic, be it SARS or any other infection. Preparing for the next outbreak requires renewing and strengthening the public health infrastructure. Many epidemiologists and other public health specialists are needed. A better surveillance and response system needs to be put in place, including stronger links between national, regional and global structures. And governments need to invest more in hospital infection control. 'SARS is teaching us many lessons,' Brundtland said. 'Now we need to translate these lessons into action. We may not have much time, and we need to use it wisely.'" Excerpt from *L'epidemia di Sars è contenuta in tutto il mondo. Comunicato dell'Organizzazione Mondiale della Sanità*, July 5, 2003 <https://www.epicentro.iss.it/focus/sars/sars-fine> (last access: November 15th, 2021).

20   Thomas Abraham, *Twenty-first Century Plague: The Story of SARS* (Baltimore MD: Johns Hopkins University Press, 2005).

21   *Prix Galien Italia 2021 a vaccino anti-Ebola Msd. Menzione speciale per trattamento Hiv in pazienti adulti*, Adnkronos, 2 November 2021 <https://www.adnkronos.com/prix-galien-italia-2021-a-vaccino-anti-ebola-msd_5bMiwGBlPUpg8esXTb2uss> (last access: November 15th, 2021).

22   *Ebola: primo caso in Costa d'Avorio, una 18enne in arrivo dalla Guinea. Oms: "Estremamente preoccupante"*, La Repubblica, 15 August, 2021, <https://www.repubblica.it/esteri/2021/08/15/news/ebola_primo_caso_in_costa_d_avorio_una_18enne_in_arrivo_dalla_guinea-314071565/> (last access: November 15th, 2021).

23   *Epidemia da virus Ebola 2014-2016* <https://www.epicentro.iss.it/ebola/epidemia-africa-2014> latest updated August 1st, 2019 (last access: November 15th, 2021).

a *Newsweek* cover title of May 5th, 2003 claimed.[24] In this case, the choice of iconography was very impactful: a health worker with a mask, because the magazine wanted to follow the narrative[25] of the previous avian influenza H10N3, which frightened us some years ago and is still found today.[26]

There is much literature that illuminates surveys of findings from the epidemic, along with assessments of what might be needed in order to contain any future outbreaks of SARS or other emerging infections. This is why I am wondering if during that time people changed their habits, since maybe it could be useful to keep that memory in order to build the passage from an unexpected danger to a 'risk-we-can-live-with'. This book is an attempt to find ways to avoid experiencing pandemics as the worst trauma of our lives: maybe 'risk-we-can-live-with' only involves considering virus pandemics a natural risk of our contemporary societies, a risk we should learn how to live with.

In the last ten years, we had the time to prepare for a future of pandemics, like the inhabitants of volcanic lands who are supposed to be ready, at least psychologically, for the next volcanic event. In fact, it is a rather common observation that shared habits in any specific place were supposed to be ultimately generated in reaction to a natural risk and/or to its threat. They can be generated by maintaining memory of how to adapt to the risk through story-telling or by certain behaviours which enable flexible responses, that can be considered long-term outcomes of living with disasters.[27]

The result of neglecting to analyse what happened to our habits during past epidemics is that, suddenly, in 2020, we experienced once again the disruption of our habits, an experience of laceration for many individuals like the main frame of the book argues.

---

24   *SARS: What You need to know – the New Age of Epidemics*, Newsweek, 5 May 2003. Stacey Knobler and others (ed. by), Institute of Medicine (US) Forum on Microbial Threats. *Learning from SARS Preparing for the Next Disease Outbreak* (Washington, DC: National Academies Press, 2004).

25   Robert Peckham, *Epidemics in Modern Asia (New Approaches to Asian History)* (Cambridge: Cambridge University Press, 2016), p. 294.

26   *Aviaria nel Veronese, una ventina i focolai*, Sky TG24 News-Veneto, November 9, 2021 <https://tg24.sky.it/venezia/2021/11/09/aviaria-nel-veronese-una-ventina-i-focolai> (last access: November 15th, 2021).

27   Robin Torrence and John Grattan, *Natural Disasters and Cultural Change* (London, New York: Routledge, 2002), p. 16. More focused on environmental disasters: Kate Rigby, *Dancing with Disaster. Environmental Histories, Narratives, and Ethics for Perilous Times* (Charlottesville: University of Virginia Press, 2015).

In respect to the great organizational inconveniences, just to suggest one instance, I wonder if the force of our habit to physically go to school, where teachers and students could be in the same room, influenced the delay in building the digital infrastructure for remote learning, which has been a plan in Italy for at least ten years.

On the other hand, maybe facing virus epidemics again forces us to bring back old habits from previous pandemics, like the digging of mass graves we saw in New York during this COVID-19 pandemic. Hart Island might be the largest cemetery for victims of the AIDS pandemic, according to the city council, but before it was the same for the yellow fever and tuberculosis outbreaks of the nineteenth century and for the victims of the great flu pandemic of 1918 too.[28]

Is it that we did something wrong in the transmission of knowledge about pandemics? Or is it that once the virus becomes weaker or a vaccine is discovered (and the fear is diminished), the mechanism of habit proves to be in many ways similar to the mechanisms of nature, reiterating the uniformity of its functioning? We are forced to admit that our collective habits represent primary points of reference in life, so we also have developed some mechanisms to defend them. Of course, if the new habits are not maintained for long enough, the old ones will reestablish themselves. Or perhaps, as in the orbital motion of celestial bodies, after a period of disruption, the forces at play could pull habits back into their original trajectory. As the Latin etymology of the word "revolution" suggests, *revolvere* is a turning back, a return to the starting point.

One of the aims of this book is to elaborate a true culture of pandemic risk. It could mean, for example, that minimizing physical contact will be the rule in the future and that we will develop a system of communication by videoconferencing where, without being able to interpret our movements in space and our sense of smell, we will still communicate efficiently.

As populations grow in the shadow of the volcano, we should adapt our habits to the risk of another pandemic. Only with habits compatible with the management of pandemics can we continue to live on this planet, which we should look at, in its entirety, as our own volcanic risk territory.

---

28   Elyse Samuels and Adriana Usero, *'New York City's family tomb': The sad history of Hart Island. Coronavirus has created a grim new reality at the nation's largest mass grave*, Washington Post, 27 April 2020 <https://www.washingtonpost.com/history/2020/04/27/hart-island-mass-grave-coronavirus-burials/> (last access: November 15th, 2021).

BERNADETTE BENSAUDE-VINCENT
TIME OF CRISIS OR CRISIS OF TIME?

Health crisis, financial crisis, economic crisis, political crisis, ecological crisis, climate crisis, personal crisis... So diverse and frequent are the crises that we come to wonder what is not in crisis! Crisis seems to be chronic, a permanent morbid state. The newspapers report day after day, year after year, all the damages that hit our societies and shake the planet. However, crisis cannot be a permanent condition. It is an oxymoron. Etymologically, a crisis (from the Greek verb *crinô*: judge, decide) is defined as a moment of decision that cuts off the passage of time. Critical is the moment when a difficult decision (or difficult decisions) must be made. In medicine, the crisis refers to the turning point of a disease, a decisive stage leading to recovery or death. If crisis becomes a normal, ordinary condition, isn't it the sign that there is something wrong with our familiar notion of a uniform timeline broken by critical episodes or disruptions? At least, it invites some reflections on our way of thinking and living time.

To begin with, it is useful to note that our experience of time is shaped by a priori categories that Immanuel Kant embedded in the transcendental ego, though they appear to be a socio-historical construction. French sociologist Émile Durkheim convincingly argued that it is a social framework resulting from continuous efforts for synchronizing social activities and representing events.[1] Our chronological framework has been gradually constructed over the centuries through the convergence of infrastructures built up by religion (calendars and almanacs), technology (sundials and clocks), society (schedules, timetables, and hourly wages), and science (units and standards).[2] The western dominant view of time is a line, stretched between a beginning and an end, the present being just a transition between the past

---

1   Émile Durkheim, *Les formes élémentaires de la vie religieuse,* 1912. On the historical construction of this framework see Krzysztof Pomian, *L'ordre du temps* (Paris: Gallimard, 1984).

2   E.P. Thompson, 'Time, work-discipline and industrial capitalism', *Past and Present,* 38 (1967): 56-97. Helga Nowotny, *Time. The Modern and PostModern*

and the future, a simple passage point.[3] This framework constitutes the order of time, in the dual sense of the term "order" as an established system or arrangement of things and as an authoritative prescription to be obeyed.

> No one doubts that an *order of time* exists—or rather, that orders of time exist which vary with time and place… For a society's relations to time hardly seem open to discussion or negotiation. The term "order" implies at once succession and command: the times (in the plural) dictate or defy, time avenges wrongs, it restores order following a disruption, or sees justice done.[4]

The modern order of time is typically epitomized by the 'arrow of progress'. The future operates on the present as "horizon of expectation".[5] Not only does it make sense of the present and the past but it is the promise to enlarge our view and transcend the present limits. This future-oriented notion of time is so deeply rooted in our culture that the arrow tends towards a catastrophe as soon as faith in progress wavers.

Although it may seem extremely difficult to get out of this pre-existing framework, it is worth considering what the recent disruptions of our ordinary regime of temporality can teach us. Based on lessons drawn from the health and environmental crises, the paper first suggests that they result from a conflict of temporalities and consequently challenge the notion of a single universal timeline. It then argues that the current focus on the global phenomenon of acceleration as responsible for the climate crisis and the beginning of the Anthropocene is missing the point because it does not question the western supremacy of a chronological view of time. In a third section the paper ventures the alternative notion of timescapes composing multiple intersecting and interdependent timelines.

1. *Lessons from the recent crises*

Over the past year, many people noted that the Covid-19 crisis acted as an indicator of problems that went unnoticed because of our

---

Experience, trans. by Neville Plaice (Cambridge: Polity Press, 1994). Ken Birth, *Objects of Time* (London: Palgrave McMillan, 2012).

3   François Jullien, *Du Temps. Eléments d'une philosophie du vivre* (Paris: Grasset, 2001). François Hartog, *Chronos; L'Occident aux prises avec le temps* (Paris: Gallimard, 2020).

4   François Hartog, *Regimes of Historicity, European Perspective*, trans. by Saskia Brown (New York: Columbia University Press, 2015), p. 1.

5   Reinhart Koselleck, *Futures Past* (Boston: MIT Press, 1985).

habitus and mind-sets. For instance, the lockdown suddenly revealed the vital importance of invisible workers such as caregivers, nurses, farmers, truck drivers, garbage collectors, cashiers, teachers. Without them the entire social system would have collapsed. Although they are indispensable, they get lower wages than many other workers. Social injustice usually concealed by our system of values jumped out during the crisis.

As individuals, we quickly realized that we had to forget about our work trip, holidays or theatre play. Our habit of planning, of organizing time has been suddenly disrupted. Setting goals and looking to the future became helpless because of too many uncertainties. So we better had to adjust to the circumstances and invent creative ways of handling the present situation.

We also learnt that the transmission rate of the virus would rule our life, limit our freedom of movement and the prospect of economic growth. A tiny virus, made of a few RNA molecules, had the power to stop air traffic, oil refineries, industrial production. In a few months it managed to reduce the emissions of greenhouse gas, a goal that the clever experts of IPP and the annual Conventions of Parties for Climate could never reach despite years of efforts. We also quickly learn that Sars-Cov 2 virus has its own lifestyle as a parasite that flourishes as long as it finds host organisms and thwarts resistance by mutating. Due to globalisation, its inexorable trajectory is entangled with the lifeline of billions of humans.

Thus the virus acts as a chemical analyser of these different timelines, and forces us to reconsider their composition. We are learning that we have to pay attention to the life trajectories of 'infinitesimal beings' — viruses, bacteria, plants, insects and others — that populate the planet. These beings that are considered 'harmful' or undesirable have their own time, their own agenda, their own right to exist. The challenge is to adapt our own plans of development to their own growth and to manage a coexistence of the fast tempo of beings that thrive by contagion with the beats of political time, economic growth, and social life.

The climate crisis has already undermined the familiar scheme of the arrow of time oriented towards a better future. It is not just because it brings about the perspective of a potential collapse of civilisation — progress or catastrophe do not radically challenge the future-oriented view of time. Techno-progressism and collapsism converge to maintain a teleogical view of time as aiming at a goal.

Since a few decades we have been experiencing the intrusion of Gaïa in our history, through heat waves, droughts, floods and hurricanes.[6] Our immoderate consumption of fossil resources has set off an incontrollable disruption of the cycles of carbon that regulate the temperature on the surface of the earth. The planet is responding to our quest for more comfort, faster mobility, and instant communication, thus questioning the dogma of economic growth through mass production and consumption. The concept of Anthropocene, the geological epoch when human activities change the course of bio-physical phenomena on the earth at a global scale, brought to light a clash between our short-term history counted in tens or hundreds years and the earth history counted in billions of years. This grand narrative widely spread in academic circles and popular media suggests that the arrow of time epitomizing social and technological progress interferes with the deep time of the earth.

To summarize the lessons from the current crises: What we call crisis appears as a conflict of timelines. Crises display conflicting temporalities that force us to experience otherness, to realize that nature is not an externality that we can exploit and submit. It is home not only to us but to billions of beings as well who have a lifetime of their own that interferes with our plans and activities. Crises teach us the contingency of our history marked by episodes of contagion and climate changes.

2. *Conflicts of tempos or rhythms?*

How are we to understand the notion of clashing temporalities? As music has an intimate connection to time, it provides a helpful distinction between tempo and rhythm. While the tempo is defined by speed, the rhythm makes a pattern made of sounds and silence. The tempo is a quantitative notion measured by the metronome, the rhythm is a qualitative way of structuring time. The 3-beat Viennese waltz can be played *allegro*: poom pam pam. *Adagio*: p o o m p a m p a m. Same rhythm, different tempos. Waltz is not the unique dance on the earth: rock, calypso, tango… afford various *rhythms*, various *patterns* of time, not just different speeds.

Anthropocene scientists describe the climate disruption as the result of clashing tempos. It is due to the speed of human development. Humans have been burning in two hundred years fossil resources that took billions

---

6   Isabelle Stengers, *In Catastrophic Times, Resisting the Coming Barabary*, trans. by Andrew Goffey (London: Open Humanities Press, 2015).

of years to grow in the underground. It is a clash between the geological and the historical scales rather than a clash of heterogeneous temporalities. Based on quantitative data, a 'great acceleration' is pointed as the cause of the Anthropocene. A series of graphs (Fig. 1) displaying the exponentials curves of socio-economic data (like population growth, economic growth, transports…) and Earth System trends (like the concentration of greenhouse gases, surface temperature, acidification of oceans).[7]

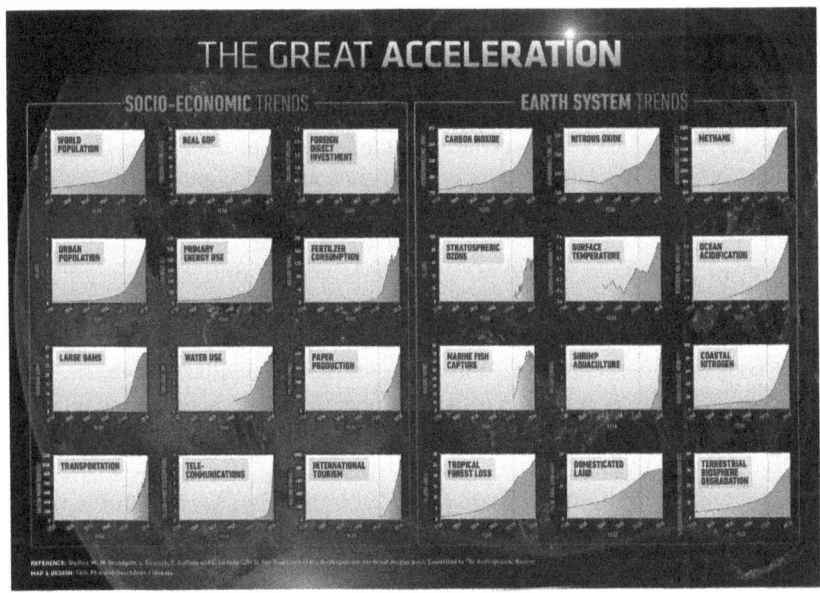

Fig. 1: The Great Acceleration. Source igbp.net

The remarkable parallelism of the curves of socio-economic and Earth system indicators is the crux of the proof. Although scientists admit that correlation does not entail causation, they conclude that this parallelism provides a good amount of evidence of human-driven changes to the Earth System. So the environmental crisis is said to result from the sharp exponential curve in the demographic and economic growth over the past

---

7   W. Steffen, W. Broadgate, L. Deutsch, O. Gaffmeny, C. Ludwig, 'The trajectory of the Anthropocene: The Great Acceleration'; *The Anthropocene Review*, 2, 2015(1), 81-98.

century that disrupted the biophysical cycle of carbon. Indeed the idea that accelerated paces of changes are responsible for a crisis is intuitive. It is all the most convincing that it resonates with the diagnosis of cultural crisis made by social scientists. Harmut Rosa in particular, convincingly argued that the accelerated pace of technological changes brings about social instability and urgency, thus generating personal and social crises as well as political crises.[8]

Nevertheless the climate crisis is not just the result of the accelerated space of demographic and economic growth. This simplistic view overlooks conflicts in the complex dynamics involving multiple heterogeneous rhythms. Not only this dynamic involves the cycles of carbon, nitrogen and oxygen but carbon itself, the bad guy of the Anthropocene, has various cycles. The most familiar is the carbon life cycle: animals burn carbon (calories), release CO_2 in respiration, which is then broken down by plants in photosynthesis, releasing oxygen. But carbon trading rather refers to the carbon cycle regulated by temperature (CO_2 absorbed by soil and oceans) as well as to the geological carbon cycle: on the scale of one million years, the CO_2 released by volcanic eruptions or underwater sources is sequestered in the form of calcium carbonate in sedimentary rocks. These rocks in turn are dissolved by river water, then by ocean water, which traps carbon, and later on by living organisms with the emergence of photosynthesis. All these cycles are operating together, each one on its own rhythm and tempo, thus generating cooperative or antagonistic and non-linear effects on the Earth system. As climate scientist David Archer explains, while the carbon life cycle has usually a stabilizing effect, the global cycle, controlled by temperature, has a destabilizing effect. It works in the opposite direction to the geological carbon cycle, which functions like a thermostat for the planet.

> The funny thing about the carbon cycle is that the same carbon-cycle machinery both stabilizes the climate (on million-year time scales) and perturbs it (on glacial cycle time scales), as if the carbon cycle were fighting with itself. It would be analogous to some erratic fault in the furnace, driving the house to warm up and cool down, while the thermostat tries to control the temperature of the house by regulating the furnace as best it can. Time to call the furnace guy![9]

---

8   Harmut Rosa, *Social Acceleration: A New Theory of Modernity*, trans. by Jonathan Trejo-Mathy (New York: Columbia University Press 2010); Judy Wacjman, *Pressed for Time: The Acceleration of Life in Digital Capitalism* (Chicago: The University of Chicago Press, 2014).

9   David Archer, *The Global Carbon Cycle* (Princeton; Oxford: Princeton University Press, 2010), p. 15.

The discrepancy of temporal rhythms is also pronounced in the living world. The on-going pandemic can be experienced and described as the confrontation between two life strategies: fitness against robustness. Unlike complex organisms, virus, bacteria and other microbes function flawlessly with a minimum of genome, they do not waste time and energy to refine their structure. In 24 hours, you get thirty generations of bacteria, whereas it takes about a thousand years to have thirty generations of humans. Microbes are always in a hurry, they don't wait years before procreating, reproduce at a rapid rate, eat all available resources and then die. They adapt to all environments through fast and repeated mutations, whereas the evolution of mammals goes slower and on quite different rhythms. The challenge is therefore to learn how to deal with a web of different timelines: that of the virus, its diffusion and (rather unpredictable) mutations, the pace that health systems can sustain, the beats of political time, economic time, social life and individual projects.

In brief, the conflicts of temporalities are not just due to a collusion between the various timescales of the chronological time. They clearly point to multiple heterogeneous temporal trajectories that do not necessarily converge in the same direction.

3. *From timescales to timescapes*

The discourses about the "great acceleration" focus exclusively on the clash of tempos because they rely on the chronological framework covering all events from the origin of the universe to the present and future climate. This universal and homogeneous timeline divided in intervals by factors of ten, based on the assumption of scale invariance, affords a Grand Narrative in which humans (*Anthropos*) feature as a tragic Promethean hero. Not only the legitimacy of the notion of one single unilinear time displaying a spectrum of timescales defined in powers of ten is not challenged, but it seems more relevant than ever. Whatever the date of the beginning of the Anthropocene, the hypothesis of a geological epoch determined by human activities reinforces the relevance of a unique timeline aligning cosmological and historical events.

Indeed making all times amenable to the measure of the powers of ten along a single line is a remarkable achievement allowing to measure the time of all natural phenomena from the disintegration of sub-atomic particles in the fraction of a second with 15 decimals to the age of the universe in billions of years. Still this all-encompassing uniform and homogeneous time jumping over factors of ten from cosmological to geological, biological, cultural and historical timescales overlooks the heterogeneity of temporal regimes that resurfaces in times of crisis. It ignores the diversity of cycles and the complex interactions between the temporal trajectories of the various components of the Earth System in order to make all times commensurable.

Moreover this great scientific achievement relies on a tacit (and questionable assumption). To embrace in a single glimpse the entire landscape from the Big Bang to nowadays and the near future you have to sit in a distance from the earth. To take a vista from outside the earth like the image of the Blue Marble of the planet earth viewed from satellites. Such a global view implies an observer outside of time, escaping from our earth-bound condition. In Bruno Latour's terms, it is not accessible to 'earthlings', to humans belonging to the earth, insiders and no longer outsiders looking at nature from nowhere.[10] This tacit assumption of extra-territoriality or extra-temporality in keeping with the modern view of humans emancipated from nature, is incompatible with the shock generated by the very idea of the Anthropocene: that we humans are integral part of nature, entangled with Earth history. In other terms, the uniform, and homogeneous, chronological timeline affords a bird's eye view at the expense of blindness on the variety and heterogeneity of times in nature and culture.[11]

Since the entanglement between multiple heterogeneous timelines becomes clearly visible in times of crisis, it may be helpful to shift from the overarching image of timescales to the metaphor of timescapes. Unlike the series of periods of time fitting together wisely like Russian dolls, let us imagine a dense landscape of coexisting and intersecting timelines.

The timescape metaphor used by historian Barbara Adam extends the landscape perspective to the dimension of time to pay attention to the entanglement of physical and cultural temporalities.[12] A timescape is constituted by anthropogenic and natural beings in interaction that make up multiscale and complex arrangements. Adam insists that humans

---

10   Bruno Latour, *Où atterrir. Comment s'orienter en politique* (Paris: La découverte, 2017).
11   On the multiple times in nature see Christophe Bouton, Philippe Huneman eds., *Time in Nature and the Nature of Time* (Boston Studies in the Philosophy of Science, Springer, 2017). On the multiple times in culture see Jérôme Baschet, *Défaire la tyrannie du présent* (Paris: La découverte, 2018).
12   Barbara Adam, *Timescapes of Modernity. The environment and Invisible Hazards* (London: Routledge, 1998), p. 9.

cannot embrace time without simultaneously encompassing space and matter—that is, without embodying it in a specific and unique context. Due to the entanglement of spatial and temporal dimensions a *landscape* is altogether a *timescape*. Timescaping the so-called successive phases of nature "deep time" and of cultural history is an alternative way of knowing and experiencing the world we live in.

It is also a good exercise to untie the close association between progress and technology fuelled by the metaphor of the time arrow. Thinking in terms of timescapes rather than timescales opens up a window on the temporalities of things we interact with and the interdependencies created by technological choices. The global health crisis due to Sars-Cov2 exemplifies the need to take into account multiple regimes of temporality. Throughout the twentieth century the fight against microbes with antibiotics fuelled the arrow of progress. The invention of antibiotics provided the evidence of the emancipation of humans from nature and instantiated progress through decoupling. But with the increasing resistance to antibiotics and the experience of a global contamination of billions of humans, we discover a quite different figure of time: contagion brings forward a time of contingency that leads nowhere, neither to a radiant future nor to a global collapse.

To sum up the on-going climate disruptions, extinction of biodiversity, and global pandemic result from conflicting temporal rhythms as much as from the acceleration of the tempo of changes. They challenge the supremacy of the chronological paradigm of Anthropocene discourses and its underlying assumption of humans as outside observers of the universal timeflow. This universal scalability appears as a device that allows domination but ultimately brings about ecological destruction and social unstability. Times of crisis can be experienced as opportunities to open the eyes on the things around us with time trajectories of their own and to try to compose timescapes of billions of entangled trajectories composing ramifying webs.

MIMESIS GROUP
www.mimesis-group.com

MIMESIS INTERNATIONAL
www.mimesisinternational.com
info@mimesisinternational.com

MIMESIS EDIZIONI
www.mimesisedizioni.it
mimesis@mimesisedizioni.it

ÉDITIONS MIMÉSIS
www.editionsmimesis.fr
info@editionsmimesis.fr

MIMESIS COMMUNICATION
www.mim-c.net

MIMESIS EU
www.mim-eu.com

Printed by
Puntoweb s.r.l. – Ariccia (RM)
July 2022